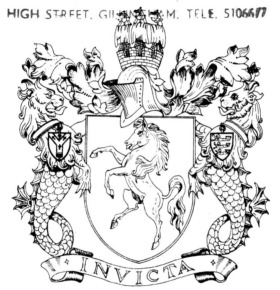

What would the world be, once bereft
Of wet and wildness? Let them be left
O let them be left, wildness and wet;
Long live the weeds and the Wilderness yet.

GERARD MANLEY HOPKINS: Inversnaid

BIKE
and
HIKE

Sixty Tours
around Great Britain
and Ireland

by
J. SYDNEY JONES

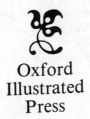

Oxford
Illustrated
Press

The publishers gratefully acknowledge: M. B. Yeats, Miss Ann Yeats and the Macmillan Company of London and Basingstoke, for permission to quote from *The Lake Isle of Innisfree*; the Society of Authors and Literary Representatives of the estate of John Masefield for permission to quote from *Roadways*; and George Allen and Unwin for permission to quote from *The Road Goes Ever On* by J. R. R. Tolkien.

ISBN 0 902280 45 7

© J. Sydney Jones, Oxford Illustrated Press, 1977

Oxford Illustrated Press, Shelley Close, Risinghurst, Oxford

Filmset by Malvern Typesetting Services Limited.

 Printed on Cyclone recycled paper

Printed and bound by Richard Clay (The Chaucer Press) Limited, Bungay, Suffolk

Contents

ROUTE GUIDES

FOR LINDA

Introduction

*To see a World in a grain of Sand
And a Heaven in a Wild Flower,
Hold Infinity in the palm of your hand
And Eternity in an hour.*

WILLIAM BLAKE: Auguries of Innocence

There is nothing exclusive about biking or hiking: the will to do it is the primary ingredient. I myself am not what would classically be called a biker: I do not walk around bow-legged in Spandex shorts, with thigh muscles rippling and hands covered in kid racing gloves, a Peugeot racing cap tucked jauntily on the back of my head; neither do I strut the streets in Dachstein boots and corduroy plus-fours. I am a writer: I enjoy travel and like to know that I have *been* somewhere when I travel—to feel a spirit of place. Biking, hiking and camping out are some of the few remaining ways of seeing the essence of places. You do not insulate yourself on a bike or on foot; you become part of the countryside; you experience the country to the full through a flood of sense input through scents and sounds that would never reach you in the womb of a coach or car.

In a world grown smaller with the jet, the way out, for those who still desire adventure and who are looking for something different is not further and further west, or deeper and deeper into space; but slower and slower through the places that they think they already know.

I began this introduction with a quotation from William Blake, which is, I think, appropriate; there is a sense of timelessness in such ordinary physical activities as biking and hiking—there is a Zen-ness to riding a bike through quiet countryside, or walking over dew-fresh ground. There are worlds within worlds when time is not measured in miles, but in feet per hour. There is no better place to look for the "World in a grain of Sand", than in the British Isles; there is everything for every kind of traveller: history and culture, great art and architecture, pastoral scenery and wilderness, and lovely villages; and the plethora of backroads and well-marked footpaths enable you to get to all these things unhassled, using your body and mind together to become much more than an "if-this-is-Monday-it-must-be-London" tourist.

Travel is very expensive. Public transport depends on oil and Britain has not been an exception to the world-wide inflation in oil prices. By biking and hiking and staying at night in a hostel or pleasant Bed and Breakfast, or sleeping under the heavens, the traveller can live reasonably and not always have to be counting pennies. Everyone travels on a budget, and although there are expenses for the biker or hiker, they are usually less than those of the ordinary tourist; and the major expenditure, on a bike or camping gear, occurs only once.

Coupled with the expense of ordinary travel is another fact: Europe has seen a terrific flood of tourists in the last decade; a sea of denim has poured over Britain and the continent and tourist traps, worse than a Disney nightmare, have sprung up in the most and least obvious places. It sounds bad, and in the high season it can be; but the high season, from May to September, especially the months of July and August, is the time when most people can travel. Unfortunately, the plans people make depend not on when they want to carry them out, but on when they can; and if you plan to be out-of-doors biking and hiking, the best months weather-wise are the high season months.

Happily, it is still easy to get away from the holiday crowds on a bike or a footpath. While other tourists are fighting the traffic inside stuffy cars or buses, or are paying exorbitant fares on trains, you can be buzzing along a quiet country lane, smelling the newly-cut hay and listening to bird song, content to travel thirty to fifty miles a day. You can stop beside fresh streams for lunch and sleep under the stars, while others are waiting in queues at Wimpy Bars and hunting frantically for already over-crowded accommodation. To travel under your own steam is to be self-contained: a traveller who has tent and sleeping bag, a gas burner and pots, needs only a plot of ground to sleep on at night, and there is a real sense of freedom in that.

Biking or hiking are two ways to escape from the constant companionship of crowds of high season tourists, while still visiting many of the typical tourist haunts. The routes in this book go through some very obvious tourist areas, such as Shakespeare country, but they take you along quiet lanes and footpaths away from the hordes and the traffic and the coach tour routes.

I like the out-of-doors, but do not eschew the luxury of a bed or a good beer, nor the comfort of a compartment on the occasional train. I bike and hike not to torture myself, but because biking and hiking have a comfort and ease all their own. All sorts of people bike on all sorts of bikes. Out of some masochistic frenzy of journalistic objectivity, just to see if any bike would do, I pedalled a 28-inch, fat-wheeled Raleigh over many of the routes in this book, and it was OK—especially downhill.

It helps to be in good physical shape if you are going to bike from thirty to fifty miles a day. But do not let flabbiness, smokers cough and general ennui be a hindrance. My biking partner on these routes was a twenty-eight year old woman who had not even seen a bike for ten years; she had lost the habit of physical exercise and, in short, did not think she had a snowball's chance in hell of completing a prolonged biking journey—alive. However, at the end of our tour we were able to do the Snowdonia region of Wales, biking up long, steep gradients through some of the roughest biking country in Britain. It was very hard work but terrifically exhilarating, especially after we had reached the summit of the range and could sail along a wide mountain plateau three thousand feet up.

This is not to say biking or hiking is easy. If you are in good physical shape you will probably be able to cover thirty miles a day on a bike, and ten to fifteen miles on foot. If you are not at all fit, you will have to take it slowly at first and there will be a couple of weeks of sore thigh muscles and aching feet; but biking and hiking will *get* you into shape. However, it is important to know your own limitations, and I will give some guidance with regard to this as I describe the routes themselves.

Many people will want to combine hiking and biking on their travels. I recommend that they do this to prevent either activity losing its novelty, and to allow the body to use different muscles, giving some a rest and breaking in others. Switching back and forth between foot and bike is especially important for those who are just starting to get into shape. You will find that after about three consecutive days of biking you just do not have the energy needed for a fourth day. Those thirty or so miles seem to stretch out in front of you forever, every breeze is a 50 mph headwind, and biking is sheer torture. Those are the days when alternative hiking routes come in handy, and there are always plenty of pubs!

Writing a book about biking and hiking in Britain is no small task. There are over 121,000 square miles, and the possibilities for getting out into the countryside on back roads and footpaths are phenomenal. In England alone there are over 100,000 miles of footpath. More than sixty biking and hiking routes form the core of this book, and in selecting them I have tried to steer that impossible middle course, to provide sufficient routes of varying difficulty to suit both the beginner and the real afficionado. There are a few instances when I could not restrain myself from giving some names of lodgings, teashops or pubs of which I have particularly fond memories, but this is the exception; that sort of discovery is up to each traveller. In most cases I just indicate the towns and cities where lodging can be found.

ONE
The Ten Touring Areas

Still round the corner there may wait
A new road or a secret gate,
And though we pass them by today,
Tomorrow we may come this way
And take the hidden paths that run
Towards the Moon or to the Sun.

J. R. R. TOLKIEN: The Road Goes Ever On

I have divided Britain and Southern Ireland into ten touring areas, with about six biking and hiking routes in each area. You may want to do all or only part of the tours, though they are arranged in a clockwise sequence as if you were doing a grand tour. Some tours are arranged around themes such as archaeology and history, literature and authors, cathedrals and brass rubbing; there is even a long pub crawl of a tour through East Anglia. Other tours are non-thematic and just take you through lovely countryside with no particular destination.

The South-East of England

This is an area of rolling hills and downs and open farmland which is sometimes referred to as the "Garden of England". It is more heavily populated than any other touring area, but it is still lovely and there are places where you can get away from the crowds. Both Canterbury, with its associations of Thomas Beckett, and Winchester, are fine cathedral cities. There are also lovely castles, notably Arundel. The Isle of Wight should be avoided during the high season when all London is day-tripping there; but it is a great place out of season, even up until mid-June. The South Coast is not much to speak of as it is very built up with many miniature Brightons, though even that can be fun for a time.

There is one long bike route across the South-East from Canterbury to Winchester, passing through many little villages with ancient churches and good opportunities for brass-rubbing. A route through the New Forest and on the Isle of Wight will introduce the traveller to two ardent avocations of every Edwardian Englishman: bird-watching and fossil-hunting.

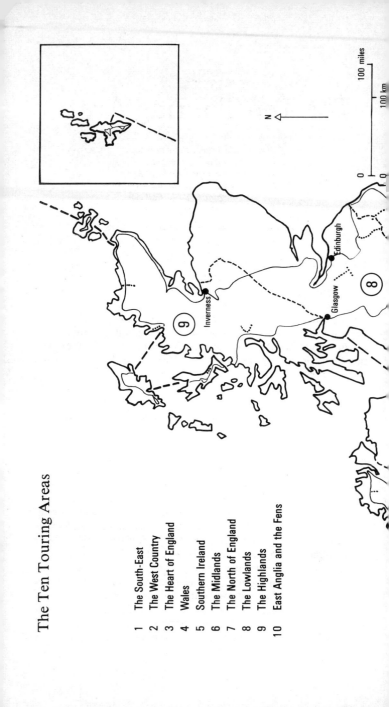

The Ten Touring Areas

1 The South-East
2 The West Country
3 The Heart of England
4 Wales
5 Southern Ireland
6 The Midlands
7 The North of England
8 The Lowlands
9 The Highlands
10 East Anglia and the Fens

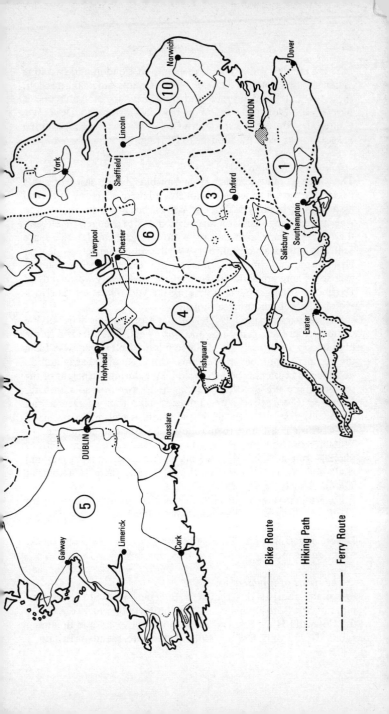

Bike Route

Hiking Path

Ferry Route

There are day walks just to the south of London and two long distance paths that are set aside by the Countryside Commission, these are both well marked and quite easy to navigate; one is part of the North Downs Way from Maidstone to Dover via Canterbury, the other is the South Downs Way which goes over the Sussex Downs from Eastbourne to Harting.

The West Country

This piece of land stretches from Salisbury in the east to Land's End in the west. The scenery is lovely and there are many historical associations, notably with King Arthur, but also with the Bronze Age and the mysteries of Avebury and Stonehenge. In Dorset, there are literary associations with Thomas Hardy; there are fantastic cathedrals at Salisbury, Wells and Exeter; cream teas in lush Devon; and, in Cornwall, some of the best coastline you will ever see. There are national parks on the vast, peaty wastelands of Dartmoor (the great, brooding Baskerville moor of Sherlock Holmes), and Exmoor to the north.

The far west, especially Devon and Cornwall, is hard biking country: there are many ups and downs and much traffic in the high season, backroads are scarce so it is difficult to get away from the bumper to bumper traffic jams. Unless you are hardy and do not mind the cars, it is best to avoid biking during the height of the season; there are excellent walking tours for this area instead. However; I do provide one immense bike tour of Devon and Cornwall, it starts at Exeter in the south, traverses Dartmoor to the Cornish coast and then follows the coast to Minehead. In Wiltshire and Somerset there is a tour of legendary and mysterious places, from sites linked with King Arthur to standing stones and chalk hill figures. To the south, in Dorset, there is a tour of Thomas Hardy's "Wessex".

For walkers there is, in Wiltshire, part of the long distance path called the Ridgeway. The South-West Peninsula Coast Path is another prodigious journey on foot around the coasts of Dorset, Devon and Cornwall. There are also two excellent, but bleak, walks on the moors.

The Heart of England

For many tourists this region *is* England, with Shakespearean plays at Stratford-upon-Avon, cozy little villages tucked away in the Cotswold Hills, and Oxford with its University and dreaming spires. If you only had a couple of weeks to spend in Britain, I would recommend you to spend them here: it is lovely country and there is much to be seen.

There is a bike tour of the Cotswolds and Shakespeare country, beginning in Oxford and leading eventually into another bike tour of the Wye Valley. Both tours offer a good mixture of scenery, history and literature: there is some terrific scenery along the River Wye, and in Herefordshire you can visit beautiful villages where the houses are built in the black-and-white half-timbered style. It is easy biking country.

For hikers there is the main portion of the Ridgeway Path that begins in Wiltshire and cuts through the Chiltern Hills to finish up just north-east of London. There are also lovely walks in the Cotswolds.

Wales

This is a beautiful country save for the gross tourist beaches in parts of the north, and the factory towns of the south. Snowdonia in the north and the Brecon Beacons to the south two national parks and lovely mountainous regions, and there is the superb coastline to the south in the Pembrokeshire National Park. The mountains in the north give way further south to moors and eventually, in the south-west, to woodland, and there are plenty of castles and isolated mountain lakes. The North tends to become crowded in the high season, especially the north-east coast which is a holiday centre for Liverpudlians and Mancunians. Wales is one of the last Celtic strongholds, and the Welsh language is still widely used.

This is adventurous biking country because of the mountains. There is a tour through Snowdonia, where you can see some of the best mountain scenery in the British Isles; another tour goes right across South Wales and includes many castles and a literary pilgrimage to the home of Dylan Thomas. For those who do not wish to venture into Wales I have included a short tour along the border country from Hereford to Chester, taking you through pretty countryside and towns where there are more of those lovely black-and-white half-timbered buildings.

Wales is also a good hiking country. There are two long distance paths: Offa's Dyke Path, which, following the ancient protective dyke built by King Offa in the eighth century AD to protect Mercia from the Welsh, stretches north to south along the Welsh/English border and is a tough path; so is the long distance coast path in Pembrokeshire, which is reminiscent of the Cornwall coast path but more difficult. There are also mountain climbs and hill walking in Snowdonia and the Brecon Beacons; you should climb Mount Snowdon—just because it is there—the ascent is not difficult; it takes about three hours to climb one of the easier paths.

Southern Ireland

Ferries leave for Ireland from the south and north of Wales. Next to Holland, Ireland is one of the best hiking countries in the world (in this context, "best" means flat). When I say Ireland, I am referring only to Southern Ireland, the Republic of Ireland. I have not included route information for Northern Ireland.

There is one long biking tour around Ireland with connecting routes between five major touring areas. The country is flat and green with peat bogs and glens; there is soda bread, and Guinness on tap; Irish is still spoken in many areas: it is a completely independent country—another world from England. The landscape can get a bit monotonous, but never the people. The biker's only enemies are the omnipresent rain and the stiff winds that blow in from the sea—and there are more coastal areas than inland areas, it seems. Some of the loveliest areas are the Wicklow Mountains, the Ring of Kerry, the Aran Islands, Connemara and Donegal. Do not miss Slieve League in County Donegal, where there is some of the most dramatic cliff scenery in the world; but do not expect too much from the over-rated County Cork.

There are walking tours in the Wicklows, Kerry, Donegal and Connemara.

The Midlands

The Midlands are not all Birmingham and smog. Some of the most magnificent country homes are here and are often on view to the public; there is also the Peak District National Park where there is good biking to the south.

For the hiker, there is the beginning of the Pennine Way which is one of the most difficult of all the long distance routes. It runs from the Peak District, along the backbone of England and over Hadrian's Wall almost into Scotland. There is good rock climbing in the Peak District, and for a different sort of challenge, try pot-holing; the Peak District is full (or should I say empty) of caves and there are many clubs which organize expeditions deep into the bowels of the earth.

The North of England

This region of beautiful and varied scenery stretches from the North Yorkshire Moors in the east to the Lake District in the West. Some areas are packed with tourists, whilst other places remain isolated and lovely. The Lake District is as crowded in the summer as Cornwall, but you must see the lakes to believe how beautiful they can be. The North offers wolds, dales and moors, Haworth and the Brontës, Hadrian's Wall and much more. It is one of my favourite touring areas. At York the Minster cathedral sits solid and forever, while the old abbeys surrounding the town are in lovely, diaphanous ruins. York is an excellent touring centre for the moors and dales and for the abbeys which surround the town. You may want to do a cathedral tour, from Durham through York to Beverly Minster, to see three of the greatest English cathedrals. The Lake District offers good biking with a route that keeps you away from the traffic as much as possible.

There is a lot of good hiking. The Pennine Way continues north into the Northumberland National Park. The Cleveland Way, another long distance path, is a hundred miles of good walking, taking the hiker past old abbeys, over moors and along the coast. The Lake District provides good hill walking and rock climbing as does the countryside around York.

(If you are doing a complete circular tour of Britain, I have assumed that you will proceed northwards through to the north-west of England into Scotland, and south from Scotland through the north-east of England to East Anglia.)

Scotland—the Lowlands

Scotland is the country of Robert Burns the poet and the tragic Mary Queen of Scots, Sir Walter Scott and Loch Lomond. The lowlands are a preview of the country further to the north, the scenery is still somewhat tame: more like England than the traditional idea of Scotland, but there is still some fine hill country and coastal scenery.

For bikers, there is a Mary Queen of Scot's tour that follows her life and times through some lovely scenery and to some splendid old castles. To the north of Edinburgh is a tour of the lochs, approaching the wild highlands.

For the hiker there are some long distance routes using ancient tracks and old Roman roads; there is also good hill-walking. The absence of public rights of way, and of inhabitants, makes cross-country walking more of an adventure here than in England.

Scotland—the Highlands and Islands

This is the rugged upland country to which Europeans flock to get away from it all. Some areas here can be more crowded than in the south, but not many, and the scenery is magnificent! The islands stretch away to the west and north so that there is always one more border, one more land mass ahead of you. The Outer Hebrides, the Isle of Skye, the Shetlands and the Orkneys are all ultimate get-away-from-it-all places for when the summer crowds begin to drive you mad. The north-west Highlands seem another world from the sheltered plains of lowland England: there are moorlands purple with the heather, there are grouse and rushing cascades of fresh mountain water. It is a lonely land when the tourists are gone: in some areas there are six people to the square mile. Be prepared for hard weather and long rides and walks far from civilization.

A bike route takes you along the north-west coastline and to many of the islands, but the complete tour is only for the hardy. It is necessary to camp unless on some days you want to pedal a hundred miles to reach accommodation.

There is hiking of the mountain variety, hill walking and good rock climbing. Be prepared for wet and cold weather.

East Anglia and the Fens

The coast of East Anglia is second only to the south of England for the deluge of tourists who arrive from London and the Midlands during the holiday season; but out of season this region is a must, and inland areas are not overcrowded even in the high season. This is low country where four hundred feet is considered a mountain. It is a biker's dream, and for this reason, especially if you are a beginner, you may want to start rather than end a tour of Britain here. East Anglia is very like Holland: it even has dykes and tulips. John Constable, the painter, was born near Ipswich and painted many scenes in the area, as did Gainsborough. The cathedrals of Ely, Norwich and Lincoln rise out of the pancake-flat landscape like Eiffel towers.

There is a bike tour of the cathedrals and Constable country combined with a pub tour on ground that is flat enough to pedal even when tipsy. There are two hikes, one on a Roman road and one on an old trackway.

These ten touring areas have been put together as if for one grand tour of the British Isles. The tours begin and end as near to London as possible because this is the main point of entry to, and departure from, Britain. To avoid backtracking, I have arranged the routes and the touring areas in a clockwise flow; so I include Ireland mid-way through the tour of England so as to make optimum use of the ferry service to and from Ireland. You may sail, for example, from South Wales to Rosslare in Ireland, and return from Dublin to Holyhead in North Wales, thus keeping to the flow of the tours and not retracing your steps. Obviously this is not the only way to tour the British Isles, some people may want to start their touring in Ireland or Scotland: the person who knows most about the kind of scenery you like, about the difficulty of grade or climb you can endure, and about how much time and energy you want to put into your tour, is yourself. You will find that once you have a good supply of maps and know what your capabilities are, that the best thing in the world is to strike off on your own; the best route-planners are human curiosity and ingenuity—never be afraid to follow either of them.

But before striking off on your own, or deciding which tour you want to do, you will need information about weather and terrain, etc. Weather is a factor which you should consider when you are deciding which areas to tour. The driest months in Ireland are May and June, in Scotland, the driest month is June, and for England and Wales, the weather is generally best in September and October. Another factor to consider is that July and August are the busiest months, so if you dislike crowds, this is the time when you want to avoid the most popular tourist areas. These areas are: Shakespeare country, the Lake District, Cornwall and Devon, the Cotswolds, Snowdonia, parts of the Scottish Highlands (especially Inverness), and the south-west of Ireland, namely Counties Cork and Kerry. This is not to say that you should not visit these regions, it is just a warning. These areas do have some of the loveliest scenery in the British Isles and you will probably want to visit one or other of them.

Warnings about the holiday season and tourist hordes are not a denunciation of "tourism" (I am one of these tourists and you will be also), but a reminder to bikers to beware, because, for them, heavily travelled roads can spell disaster; at best, it is not much fun to be forever jockeying for position with caravans and cars.

Another factor to take into account when you choose your itinerary is geography. As the south of England is the most heavily populated area in Britain (and tends to be the most touristy), routes in the south are geared more to the human than to the scenic, for example: architecture, history, literature, and beer. Whereas in the far north, in northern Scotland, in Wales and the Republic of Ireland, the tours are primarily scenic, taking you through wild and beautiful country. Between these two geographic extremes is a blend of both the scenic and the human/cultural.

I have attempted to begin one tour as close as possible to where the preceding tour leaves off, so that you can bike in between the tours. Or I have ended one tour at a point where you can catch a train to the next tour. There are some very long distances to be covered between some tours, and you could be a fairly old person by the time you have completed a grand tour of the British Isles using no public transport.

The tour descriptions are divided up arbitrarily between towns. These divisions are not necessarily a prescribed number of miles for a day, but are a logical convenience for the reader. There is no prescribed daily mileage other than that beginners should not try to do more than twenty or thirty miles at the beginning.

The letter "L" after a place-name means there is lodging, either hotel or Bed-and Breakfast "H" means a hostel; and "C" means that there is an official campsite, usually with toilet facilities. If a place does not have an "L" following, it does not necessarily mean that no lodgings exist there, just that there are none that I know of personally.

BIKE ROUTES

The biking routes in this book are not an attempt to cover the whole field of touring in Britain. There are, in Britain and Ireland, literally thousands of backroads and pathways on which to roam. However the routes in this book are a good introduction and will keep you going for many months. If you have a good supply of maps at your disposal, you can explore the countryside for yourself, and plan your own tours. You can expect to cover from twenty-five to fifty miles a day, depending on terrain and weather and past biking experience. This will help you to gauge possible B and B or hostel stops. If you join the Cyclists' Touring Club (see page 214), they will help you to plan your routes.

There is one last tip, which a Kentish woman, a veteran of forty years of hilly biking in her home county, gave to me. Do not avoid those purple areas on the map just because they are high and mountainous. In mountainous country you will see some of the most magnificent scenery in the British Isles. And besides, biking may even be easier than in those areas that merely vary in shades of green on the map, for those areas can be absurdly hilly, a constant up and down that can wear you out very quickly. Mountain areas might give you one long pull uphill and then a long ride on a mountain plateau, followed by a long, happy ride whizzing downhill into the valley. As this lady explained to me, "what's the worry? Once you're up, you're up."

THE HIKING PATH

In England, there are long distance footpaths and bridleways, national routes, with a continuous right of way for walkers—and for cyclists and horse-riders too, when the path is wide enough to be designated a bridleway. These paths allow you to make journeys lasting two weeks and more, cross country, avoiding traffic and civilization; or you may just want to use a section of a public path for a fine day's walk. The long distance paths are sign-posted with an acorn symbol:

There are now eleven such paths designated by the Countryside Commission, and nine of these eleven have been opened. Each of these paths is described in the relevant touring area, here I will list the paths and give them a difficulty rating.

The Pennine Way, Offa's Dyke Path, the Pembrokeshire Coast Path, and the Cleveland Way all pass through some lovely, but rough, mountainous country, and are for the experienced hiker. Parts of these paths are quite easy, so if you are an inexperienced walker, each of these paths offers good day-walks.

The Southwest Peninsular Coast Path is divided into four sections: Dorset, South Devon, Cornwall, and Somerset/North Devon (this last part is not yet completely open). These paths would suit the intermediate walker, someone who has had some hiking experience, but, again, there are some quite easy stretches for day-walks. Do not miss the fine scenery on the Cornwall Coast Path, especially on the west coast.

The Ridgeway Path, the South Downs Way, and the North Downs Way all provide pleasant, peaceful scenery, though not spectacular like the first four upland paths, and these could be termed easy: easy to follow and easy to hike, with many villages supplying lodging along the course of the path. Of course at points along all the long distance paths, lodging may not be easy to find either at hostels or in small town B and Bs, so camping equipment should be carried.

I have developed some shorter walks directly from the red, dotted lines on the 1:50,000 Ordnance Survey maps. Canals built in the industrial nineteenth century, and largely disused today, provide good walking opportunities along their towpaths; also old Roman roads that have not become modern highways—not to mention Hadrian's Wall. Some of the moors have ancient trackways criss-crossing them; and in the more mountainous regions such as Snowdonia, the Lake District, and the hills and mountains of Scotland, there are old and new routes for hill-walking.

The ten national parks in England and Wales all have marked trails and there are usually printed guides of these trails for sale at the park headquarters. (see page 220)

This book does not cover specialities such as rock climbing, however the best centres for that are in Snowdonia, the Lake District, the Scottish Highlands and Islands, and in County Donegal in the Republic of Ireland.

In short, there are all sorts of hikes and walks in the Isles for all sorts of people. This book is an introduction to the thousands of different walks available.

TWO
The South-East

Kent, Sir—everybody knows Kent—
apples, cherries, hops and women

CHARLES DICKENS : Pickwick Papers

In South-East England there is the rich farmland of Kent and Surrey, and the chalk cliffs at Dover; there are beautiful cathedrals and lovely little villages. The main roads are crowded during most of the year, but there are many pleasant lanes and footpaths where you can get away from the congestion and noise of the motorized world.

There are two good bike routes across the southern counties: the first takes you from one great cathedral to another, and the second shows you the contrasts between a string of seaside resorts and a nature reserve where you can do some bird-watching.

There are many good hikes in this area: two easy long distance routes across open country, as well as day-walks: one taking in Winston Churchill's home, and another along the Dover Cliffs. There are also seashore and forest trail walks.

The bike routes in the South-East are covered by maps 16 and 17 in the Ordnance Survey Quarter-Inch Series, and by maps 5, 6, 8, 9 and 10 in the Bartholomew 1:100,000 Series.

BIKING

CANTERBURY to WINCHESTER
(130 miles)

This tour takes you from one cathedral city to another via the orchards and Weald of Kent, and the downs of Sussex and

Hampshire. There are plenty of fascinating old churches, and places of historic interest. You might try your hand at brass rubbing along the route, but before setting up your paper on a likely brass, ask an official at the church for permission to take a rubbing.

Canterbury to Biddenden (27 miles)

Canterbury (LCH) is a good place to begin a tour of England, and it is only a short train or bus ride from London. See the cathedral, a massive building where Thomas Becket, an early martyr to the conflict between church and state, was killed by King Henry II's men.

From Canterbury proceed south-west on the A28, a not too busy main road, through the Canterbury suburbs, to Tharington and then to Chartham, three miles away. Orchard country begins here, so try some Kent cider or barley wine, it's powerful stuff! The thirteenth to fourteenth century church at Chartham has some fine examples of Kentish tracery, or metal grill work, in its eastern windows. There are also good brasses in the north transept. Three miles further on is Chilham (see under *Hiking*) one of the loveliest villages in Kent. Chilham Castle, a Jacobean mansion, was built in 1616, supposedly from plans by the architect Inigo Jones. Continue south-west on the A28 to Godmersham, where there is a twelfth century bas relief of St Thomas Becket, the earliest known sculpture of the saint.

Turn left at Godmersham and continue for a few miles on a minor road to the ancient little town of Wye, where there are several fine old houses, and pleasant views across the Stour Valley. Wye is the birthplace of Aphra Behn, a fascinating woman: a novelist, dramatist and spy; she was the first woman to write for the English stage and the first to be a spy; she was employed by Charles II against the Dutch. This backroad rejoins the A28 at Kempe's Corner where you turn left, and continue into Ashford (LC). This is a fairly large, and fairly busy market town, with a nice church, built on the site of a former one which is mentioned in the *Domesday Book*.

Stay on the A28 going south-west out of Ashford, through Great Chart with its many old houses and a church with good brasses; then on through quiet, pastoral countryside to the A262 for Biddenden (LC). This is a village out of the text-books with its fine half-timbered weavers' cottages, built in the fifteenth century, and its medieval Cloth Hall.

Biddenden to East Grinstead (45 miles)

Take the A262 out of Biddenden towards Sissinghurst. Harold Nicholson and Vita Sackville-West made their home here at Sissinghurst Castle, which is now open to the public. It is worth a visit as it is a fine example of an English country home with gardens.

Continue on to Goudhurst (H) and at the junction of the road to Lamberhurst, bear right for the A21 to Pembury. This part of the ride traverses an elevated ridge and gives good views. At Pembury bear left on the A263 for Royal Tunbridge Wells (L). Plain old Tunbridge Wells was dubbed Royal by a king. It was a spa, during the Regency Period, to which royalty flocked before sea-bathing became the thing to do. There is a museum of Victoriana. From Tunbridge Wells the route goes mostly along the backroads through quiet, pleasant country.

Take the A264 out of Tunbridge to Crockers Hatch Corner, then turn right on to the B2188, the Penshurst Road, and then left after a quarter of a mile on to the road for Ashurst. You follow this road through Highfields Park, Blackham, across the Edenbridge Road (five miles up the B2026), and on to Holtye Common. This road continues past Hammerwood, a two hundred year-old estate, and finally rejoins the main road at East Grinstead (C, two miles south).

East Grinstead to Petworth (32 miles)

Take the B2110 out of East Grinstead. At Whitley Hill this route joins the B2036, but after a quarter of a mile there is a right turn on to the B2110 through Balcombe Forest. From Handcross go south on the A279 for four miles and then turn right on to the A281 for Horsham (C, three miles), a medium-sized market town with the interesting thirteenth century St Mary's Church. From here you take a route that leads across rich meadows and through fine oak woods. Take the A264 out of Horsham for Five Oaks. At Broadbridge Heath you will pass Field Place where the poet Shelley was born.

Take the A29 at Five Oaks for Billinghurst where you follow the A272 to Wisborough Green, a pleasant town which was a glass-blowing centre in the Middle Ages. Continue south-west through Flexham Park—a little rise of five hundred feet—to Petworth (L); go to see the magnificent collection of pictures, and the carvings by Grinling Gibbons at Petworth House.

The South-East of England

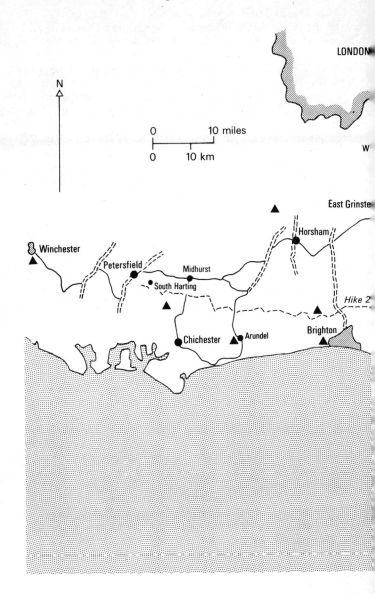

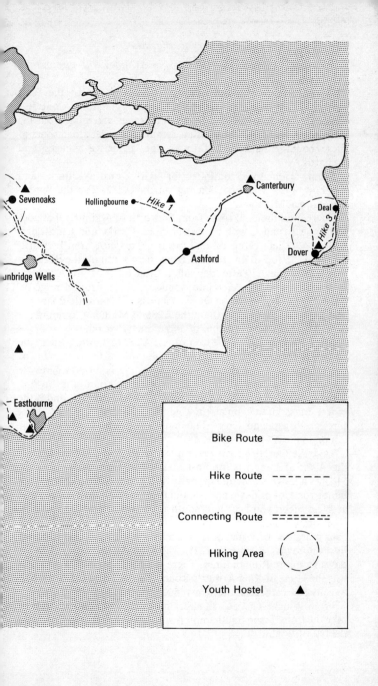

Petworth to Winchester (37 miles or 65 miles with an optional tour)

This route takes you through the pleasant valley of the West Rother. Leave Petworth on the A272 for Tillington. Along this whole stretch you will find lovely little lanes diverging from the main road, and it will be worth a detour to wander along some of these country lanes and through the attractive villages and orchards.

From Tillington continue through Cowdray Park and Eastbourne to Midhurst, staying on the A272. Try the Spread Eagle Inn at Midhurst.

There is an optional route from Petworth to Midhurst that goes south via Arundel, with its fine Norman Castle, and Chichester, with its excellent cathedral and theatre. Go south from Petworth on the A283 to Fittleworth and from there south on the B2138 to join up with the A29 after two miles. Branch left off the A29 after four miles on to the A284 into Arundel (LCH). From here go on the A259 to Chichester via Queen Victoria's "dear little Bognor"; and from Chichester, north on the A286 to Midhurst to rejoin the tour. This is a one-day detour of about thirty-five miles.

From Midhurst continue west on the A272 to Trotton where the church is famous for the brasses in the floor of the nave. One of these brasses, from the thirteenth century, is of Margaret de Camays in the dress of the period with an inscription in flowing Lombardic lettering—it is a real prize for brass-rubbers, and is the oldest brass of a woman in England. Continue on the A272 through Rogate and across the Hampshire border where you bear left on to the A3 for Petersfield (L).

Take the Langrish road west out of Petersfield and bear left off the A272 at Langrish for East and West Meon in the unspoilt Meon Valley (East Meon especially, is a good walking centre), the minor road loops down and around through both little towns, and at West Meon you bear left, south to Warmford where you turn right on to a lane which will take you back on to the A272 some four miles east of Winchester. Turn left on the A272 and continue into the town. Winchester (LH) was King Alfred's capital but it dates from pre-Roman times. There is a tradition that Winchester was the home of King Arthur's Round Table. There is a castle and a really fine cathedral; the nave is 560 feet: the longest in Europe.

From Winchester you can either bike down to Southampton or take the train. From Southampton you catch the ferry to Cowes on the Isle of Wight.

ISLE OF WIGHT and NEW FOREST TOUR
(90 miles)

The Isle of Wight is separated from the mainland only by the Solent and has little of the isolated island atmosphere that you will find in the north; but still there is something special about it: a feeling of compactness that makes it an ideal place for the biker. There are lots of spas and unfortunately much traffic also, but it can be pleasant with its Victorian associations. I have not given any routes to the east of the island, through the resorts of Ryde, Sandown and Shanklin because of heavy tourist congestion and because if you have seen one Brighton, you have seen them all. There is an optional short ride to Ventnor, the nicest and the earliest of the Victorian spas in the south.

Cowes to Yarmouth (45 miles)
Cowes, where the ferry drops you, is now the home of the Royal Yacht Club. Across the bay in East Cowes is Osborne House, the home built for Queen Victoria, and where she died in 1901: it should not be missed by any serious student of Victoriana. The state apartments and the grounds are now open to the public. Osborne is a treasure house of Victoriana: carvings, paintings, gildings; there is one whole room where everything is made out of antler!

From Cowes travel south on the A3021 for four miles to Newport. This is the county town of the Island and lies along the banks of the Medina. Proceed south from Newport on the A3020 through Rookley to Godshill, a further seven miles. Godshill is a picturesque village with thatched cottages around the church; it is popular for its cream teas.

Take a minor road south to Whitwell (HC). From here you may take a short optional route into Ventnor only three miles to the east or continue west over St Catherine's Hill and see the lighthouse that used to be one of the most powerful in the world—as powerful as 700,000,000 candles! Join the A3055 road and follow it to Chale four miles away. Follow the A3055 north from Chale along the coast past some lovely coastal scenery to Brook where you turn right, inland, on the 3041 to Carrisbrooke, eight miles away. Here you will find an excellent castle and a church with a finely carved pulpit.

Go north from Carrisbrooke on a minor road to the A3054 and turn left through Shalfleet, into Yarmouth. This is a cheery little

Isle of Wight and New Forest

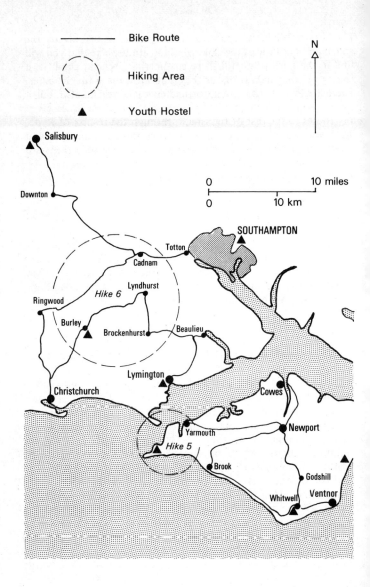

harbour town with a sixteenth century castle. From Yarmouth you can either continue on to the next tour, or take another short optional route four miles to the south-west to Alum Bay (see under *Hiking*). Alum Bay is where Marconi made his first radio transmission, but more importantly for most day-trippers to Wight, this is fossil-hunting and memento country: thousands upon thousands of tourists have filled little bottles with the twelve shades of sands from the sandstone cliffs, and still the cliffs stand (for the time being).

From Yarmouth you can catch the ferry to the mainland to begin the New Forest tour.

You can still see the white of the salt in the marshes to the south of Lymington as your ferry approaches the mainland from Yarmouth. Salt used to be big business here, but not any longer; so also was ship building, but that was in the days when the giant oaks of the New Forest supplied timber for some of the best ships in Her Majesty's Fleet. The New Forest is no longer all giant oaks. The word "forest" does not necessarily describe a wooded area: "forest" as the word is applied here means a tract of land, owned by the King, which was left uncultivated to be used as a hunting preserve; the New Forest also includes heathland. The king in this case was William the Conqueror, who set aside this area of nearly one hundred square miles for red deer. Today the New Forest is controlled by the Forestry Commission and is a preserve for all sorts of animals and plants. An interesting piece of trivia concerning the New Forest is that in days of royal landholding, privileges were granted to the commoners who lived in and around the Forest, such as grazing, limited hunting, and the right to collect firewood. Those who were granted wood rights could only collect the wood which a man could hook off with a crooked stick. From this practice comes the expression "by hook or by crook".

This bike tour (and the hiking tour of the same area) can be devoted to bird watching and flower identifying; and a couple of books—one on plants and the other on birds—might be useful for those who are interested in flora and fauna.

Lymington to Cadnam (45 miles)

The following route takes you through the heart of the Forest, but first we will take a short trip from Lymington (LH) to the east on the B3054 to Beaulieu. Here you will find the ruins of a thirteenth century monastic village. There is not much left, but the foundations can be traced and there are still some arches remaining in the cloisters; the present parish church was once the refectory of the monastery. Nearby are a brewery and a vineyard: signs of the good life which the monks must have lived. The fields to the south of the abbey are still called the Vineyard and grapes were harvested there until 1730. In the town of Beaulieu is the National Motor Museum which contains one of the finest collections of cars, motorbikes and cycles in the world.

Travel west from here on the B3055 to Brockenhurst. This is the home of the hobby horse, where a Mr Pope invented the toy that still thrills little children all over the world. This is the real beginning of the New Forest. Travel north from here on the A337 to Lyndhurst which is the main town of the area and surrounded by woods. From Lyndhurst you travel about three miles south-west on the A35 until you come to a road branching right for Burley. It is six miles in all from Lyndhurst to Burley (H), which is another good centre for walks (see under *Hiking*).

Leave Burley south-west by back lanes for Bransgore, and from there to Sopley or Winkton where you meet the B3347, on which you turn left for Christchurch, an old monastic town near the coast with a fine twelfth century church, and the Lady Chapel: both good pieces of craftsmanship. There is a memorial to Shelley in the church (the same memorial was turned down by Westminster Abbey). Continuing north on the B3347, you come, after eight miles, to Ringwood (L) which is the market town of the area, noted once solely for the knitted woollen gloves which were made there called "Ringwoods".

From Ringwood proceed back across the Forest to Cadnam, via the A31, over ground considered the loveliest in the New Forest. Cadnam (L) is the northern entrance to the Forest; some two miles south, just off the A31, left on to the narrow road going steeply to Canterton Glen, is the Rufus Stone, perhaps worth a small detour on the way to Cadnam. This stone was set up on the spot where an arrow reputedly glanced off an oak in 1100 and killed King William Rufus. You will probably hear this legend or see tourist mementoes referring to it from one end of the Forest to the other, so you can at least see where it all started.

If you want to proceed from Cadnam to the next bike tour which starts at Salisbury, you can either bike via the B3078 from Cadnam for five miles then take a right fork on to the B3080 for Downton, and from Downton take the A338 north to Salisbury, which is a sixteen mile connecting route; or, four miles east of Cadnam on the A336 is Totton where you can catch a train. (see under *Hiking*)

HIKING

THE NORTH DOWNS WAY
(43 miles)

This is just a section of the total 141 mile route across the North Downs. The forty-three miles included here have been signposted by the Kent County Council. Along part of this path you follow the broad track called the Pilgrims' Way; this track was so-called because it was one of the routes along which pilgrims travelled on their way to Canterbury to visit Thomas Becket's shrine; but this part of the Pilgrims' Way is actually much older than medieval times: it dates back to the Neolithic era, three to four thousand years ago, when this old straight track was first pounded out by Neolithic tribesmen who landed where Dover now stands and travelled on foot to the plains of Wiltshire to settle—to Stonehenge and Avebury (see next chapter). The path also passes through typical Kent orchard country and some attractive villages. Some stretches of the route are bridleway and can be used by horse-riders and cyclists.

This forty-three mile stretch of the Pilgrims' Way starts at Hollingbourne, not far south of London, and traverses the North Downs via Canterbury to Dover. The way is marked by low signstones where it leaves public roads and occasionally elsewhere. These signstones bear the words *North Downs Way*. In other places of doubt about the correct path, it is indicated by the acorn waymarker.

Maps in the Ordnance Survey 1:50,000 Series are 188, 189 and 179. The path is generally easy walking with several villages along the way where you can find accommodation.

1. Hollingbourne to Dover via Canterbury (43 miles)
From the village of Hollingbourne you begin by picking up the old Pilgrims' Way near the Pilgrims' Rest pub. You follow the ancient trackway for nine miles below the Downs; to the right is the Weald, and you continue past Harrietsham and Lenham to Charing (L). Then, still on the Pilgrims' Way, you go through Eastwell, skirting Eastwell Park, and on to Boughton Aluph. From here the path follows the Downs as they turn north and ascends Soakham Downs, continuing along the edge of Challock Forest with Godmersham Park and the river below. The path then

proceeds alongside Chilham Park to the attractive village of Chilham with its castle and lovely ancient square. After Chilham the path soon comes to the outskirts of Canterbury (LCH) and enters the town of Harbledown. You will pass through the lovely orchards which surround Canterbury. To leave Canterbury, you follow the A257 road on the east side of the town and the path leaves this road south-east to Patrixbourne and then continues by Barham Downs to the villages of Womenswold and Sibertswold. Not long after passing through Waldershare Park, the path changes direction abruptly to the south for Dover. It reaches Dover (LHC—see under *Day-Walks* in this section) by the Roman road near Connaught Park.

THE SOUTH DOWNS WAY
(80 miles)

This is probably one of the best long distance paths that you could find. It runs right across Sussex from Eastbourne in the east, to the Hampshire border in the west. It mainly follows the ridge of the South Downs and is a well marked trail, one that even those who have never hiked before can thoroughly enjoy. To hike the whole way, you would need about a week, but sections of the path can be hiked from any of several access points along the route. The eastern half of the route gives you good views over the Weald most of the way from such viewpoints as Windover Hill, Firle Beacon and Ditchling Beacon; to the south are the rolling downs and an occasional glimpse of the sea. The countryside becomes more wooded in the west and there are fewer open views, though there are good viewpoints at Rackham, Bignor Hills, Cocking Down and Harting Down.

The South Downs Way is bridleway for the entire route and is therefore open to cyclists, horse-riders and hikers. There are parts of the path where you have to walk your bike, but it is still a good bike route. Oak signs with the words *South Downs Way* mark the places where the route leaves a road or at junctions with other paths. On the open downlands there are small stone plinths with the same words. The acorn symbol is also used with these signs as well as being stencilled on walls, fences and stiles along the route. If you have any doubt about the proper path, remember that it follows the ridge of the South Downs as closely as possible.

The Ordnance Survey 1:50,000 maps for this are 197, 198, 199

or there is *Brighton and the Sussex Vale* in the Outdoor Leisure
Map Series, with a scale of 1:25,000. A useful guidebook is
published by the Eastbourne Rambling Club, called *Along the
South Downs Way,* and is available from bookshops in the area or
by post from Mr H. Comber, 28 Kinfauns Avenue, Eastbourne,
Sussex, BN22 8SS.

2. Eastbourne to the Hampshire Border (80 miles)

From the outskirts of Eastbourne (CLH), a somewhat elegant
resort of Victorian and Georgian character, you can take one of
two paths to Alfriston (LH) about fifteen miles away. The inland
path goes along the high edge of the Downs round the west of the
town as far as Willingdon Hill, then cuts north-west across the
Downs via the village of Jevington to Windhover Hill, and then
down into Alfriston in the Cuckmere Valley. The other route takes
you along the top of the cliff top around Beachy Head, but is not
suitable for horses or cyclists; take the path south-west out of
Eastbourne around Beachy Head to Burling Gap, the Seven Sisters
(seven dramatic chalk cliffs over five hundred feet high), and from
there north to Cuckmere Haven, Exceat Bridge, West Dean,
Charleston, Litlington, and into Alfriston (LH).

From Alfriston this bridleway stays close to the north-west
facing scarp of the Downs for seven miles, passing over Firle
Beacon until it comes to the Ouse Valley at Southease. From here
the path takes a wide sweep north passing just below Lewes (L),
crosses the A27 at Newmarket Inn and arrives at a point just by the
village of Plumpton.

From here the bridleway turns west again, keeping to the scarp
for six or seven miles, and passing over Ditchling Beacon to the
village of Pyecombe (Patcham LH, two miles). Here you cross the
A23 but then climb back up to the scarp at Devil's Dyke, a V-
shaped cleft in the Downs with long views over the Weald. There is
a legend which says that the devil, in an effort to stop Christianity
from spreading, began digging this trench so that the Weald would
be flooded with waters from the Channel. A woman who was
watching scared the devil away before he finished the monumental
task by holding a candle up which the Prince of Darkness mistook
for the rising sun.

Continue over Edburton Hill just west of Fulking where the
route leaves East Sussex and enters West Sussex. The route stays
on the ridge over Truleigh Hill (H), then descends to the Adur
Valley near Botolphs, crossing the A283 and then the river by the

new bridle bridge. It passes to the south of Upper Beeding, Bramber (L) and Steyning (L).

Then, west of Steyning, the path continues above Wiston Park to Chanctonbury Ring on the crest of the Downs, a magical ring of beech trees planted in 1760 around an Iron-Age hill fort. The Romans occupied the hill in the third century AD and there are the remains of Roman buildings in the centre of the ring. From the ring you descend and cross the A24 just south of Washington (L). Then, continuing by way of Highden, Kithurst, Rackham Hills and Amberley Mount, the path reaches the Arun Valley and the villages of Amberley and Houghton (L; Arundel, HL, three miles). After this comes Bury Hill where you cross the A29, and then Stane Street, a Roman Road, at Bignor. From Stane Street, the ridge of the Downs runs north to south for two miles while the path goes north-west by Burton Down and across the A285 at Littleton Farm near Upwaltham, meeting the ridge again on Woodlavington Down. From there the path continues on to Graffham and Manorfarm Downs where there are large deciduous forests.

The path crosses the A286 just south of Cocking (L) and goes by Linch Down and Diddling Hill to Philliswood Down, where it turns north-west close by Buriton Farm, to reach Pen Hill. It passes south of Beacon Hill (793 feet), or may be followed up and over that hill with a steep ascent and descent, then across Harting Downs to Tower Hill. At this point the path crosses first the B2141 and then the B2146 and follows Forty Acre Lane to the West Sussex boundary, ending at a point near Sunwood Farm, although there is a bridleway that continues into Hampshire through Queen Elizabeth Forest and crosses the A3 to Butser Hill and beyond.

For more information about accommodation along the route, write, with stamped addressed envelope included, to Mr Charles Shippam, Priory Cottage, Boxgrove, Chichester, Sussex or to the Countryside Commission. There are hostels at Portsmouth and Hindhead, but some parts of the Downs are fairly remote and it may be difficult to find lodging exactly when and where required. It is always best to have camping equipment and be sure to carry water as the river water is often unfit for drinking. Most sections of the South Downs Way are within a mile or two of bus or rail services. You reach the eastern end by Eastbourne Corporation buses. At the western end, the Southdown buses from Petersfield Station deliver you either to Buriton or South Harting. Stations near the route for access or egress are: Polgate, Lewes, Southease,

Hassocks and Amberley. Brighton, Chichester and Shoreham-by-Sea are also good connecting points for buses.

TWO DAY-WALKS in SOUTH-EAST ENGLAND

There are two good shorter walks near the first of the long distance paths, the North Downs Way; they are especially good for bikers who want a day's relief from the bike. One path goes from Deal on the coast in south-east Kent to Dover, and is one of the finest cliff walks in England, about eleven miles long. The other is a ten mile walk between Westerham and Sevenoaks, which is about twenty-five miles to the south of London, and includes two famous houses, Chartwell, Sir Winston Churchill's home, and Knole, the Sackville's Jacobean house.

Deal to Dover (11 miles)

Deal and Dover were two of the "Cinque Ports", part of a federation of twenty ports and fortresses built by Henry VIII as a defence against an invasion from Europe after the break with the Church of Rome. At Deal you can still see one of the three castles that were built here, the largest and most elaborate of all the forts built by Henry VIII. Julius Caesar landed at Deal in fifty-five BC, as, in 1170, did Thomas Becket on his return from exile. William Penn sailed from Deal in 1682 on his first voyage to America. Deal is now known for golf and sea-bathing—something of a come-down from its past associations.

From Deal take the B2057, a small back road, to Kingsdown, three miles away; here skirt the edges of the Walmer and Kingsdown Golf Links, climb over Hope Point to the Dover Patrol Monument and then down to St Margaret's Bay, another three miles. At the first bend above the cove road leading out of St Margaret's Bay there is a path leading up to a ridge and the South Foreland's Lighthouse. The route at this point runs inland in two places to skirt cliff-top coves, but otherwise runs high above the sea providing views as far as the French coastline on clear days. Continuing on, Dover harbour and castle will shortly come into view. You descend the cliffs by the Eastern Docks which is where the Boulogne car-ferry docks, and from here you can catch a bus into Dover, one mile away. This last part of the walk is about five miles.

Dover's white cliffs are the end of the chalk downs from the north. The building of Dover Castle was started in 1064 by King Harold, only two years before he was killed at Hastings; the victor of that battle, William the Conqueror, continued the building of it, as did Henry VIII who used it as one of his Cinque Ports. The castle was last used in the Second World War. It is said that you can see the history of England in stone at Dover: from the time of the old Roman port, called Dubris, to the hustle and bustle of today's busy port, Dover has been Europe's gateway to England.

Map 179 in the Ordnance Survey 1:50,000 Series should be used for this walk.

4. *Westerham to Sevenoaks (10 miles)*

You take the path from Westerham (L) which leaves from the south side of the green. It is signposted to Hosey Hill. There is an easy ascent, giving good views back toward Westerham and the North Downs. The path joins another which continues along a hedge then into a valley. At this point you join a third path which takes you up and over Hosey Common. You soon come to the Edenbridge Road where you turn right. Walk along this road for a quarter of a mile until you reach a lane signposted to Chartwell: this is the home that Sir Winston Churchill loved, his solace during those nerve-racking war days; you can still see the wall he built as a means of relaxation from the tensions of wartime. Chartwell is nothing special architecturally, but it gives good views over the Kentish Weald, and you can see the study where Churchill worked, usually standing up at a desk specially made for this purpose; there are also rooms which are full of his oil paintings. The house is open to the public on Wednesdays and Thursdays from two p.m. to six p.m. and on Saturdays and Sundays from eleven a.m. to six p.m.

The lane continues on to Mariner's where a path leads to Crockham Hill, Toys Hill, and Ide Hill and on to Sevenoaks. From Sevenoaks it is just a short walk to Knole: at the end of the High Street, opposite the parish church, the one thousand acres of Knole Park begins. Paths and a road lead to the house, which is open Wednesdays to Saturdays, ten a.m. to three-thirty p.m. There are other entrances for pedestrians at River Hill, Fawke Common, and Golden Greene.

Knole has been in the Sackville family since 1566; Vita Sackville-West was brought up here and once described the house with all its chimneys and gables, as looking more like a "medieval village" than the home of just one family. There is a fine Jacobean staircase, paintings by Van Dyck and Reynolds, and in the entrance hall there is a manuscript by Vita's friend, Virginia Woolf: the manuscript of *Orlando* which had its setting at Knole.

Ordnance Survey maps 187 and 177 in the 1:50,000 Series should be used for this walk.

WALKS ON THE ISLE OF WIGHT
and IN THE NEW FOREST

There are two more walks that correspond with bike touring areas on the Isle of Wight and in the New Forest: a one-day excursion from Yarmouth to Alum Bay and back, on the Isle of Wight; and a two-day circular walk, from Cadnam to Burley and back, in the New Forest.

5. *Yarmouth to Alum Bay to Yarmouth (12 miles)*

From Yarmouth cross the River Yar on the Norton Road going west. At Norton you will find a path leading out of the town to the south-west to Colwell Bay, and from that bay follow the coast around to the lovely Totland Bay. At the Totland Bay Hotel take the road nearest the coast for a short distance and then fork right by a path over Headon Hill (four hundred feet) to Alum Bay. The cliffs here, besides yielding twelve colours of sand, are also full of fossils as are those at Colwell Bay. Continue eastwards and fork right for Freshwater Bay. You will pass by Farringford House, which is now a hotel, but was formerly the occasional home of the poet, Tennyson, during the years 1853 to 1892. Lady Tennyson is buried in the Freshwater churchyard.

From Freshwater Bay, a road leads north to Freshwater Station and then back through Norton to Yarmouth; or a right fork before the station takes you on to the Carrisbrooke Road. Turn right on this road and go east towards Carrisbrooke for half a mile and then turn left, north on to the Thorley road and walk back to Yarmouth via Thorley.

You will need Ordnance Survey map 196 in the 1:50,000 Series for this walk.

6. *Cadnam to Burley to Cadnam (26 miles)*

From Cadnam you proceed on the B3078 for about three miles until the second turning, to Fritham. Continue south-west through Fritham on a minor road to the A31, where you turn right.

Proceed for about four miles to Picket Post where you turn left on to a minor road through Burley Street, and then by another minor road to Burley (H). (There are many good forest walks in the Burley area.) From Burley another minor road leads north-east through Burley Walk to the A35, about five miles away. Turn left, going north-east on the A35 through Bank, and turn left, north on to a small road to Emery Down. Continue north on this road and then bear right on a minor road for Newton and Minstead. Bear left at Minstead, going north to the A31. Just across the A31 at this point is another minor road leading north to the Rufus Stone (see under *Biking*). You can make a short detour to this spot or just turn right on to the A31 for Cadnam.

You will need Ordnance Survey maps 195 and 196 in the 1:50,000 Series. For further walks in this area there are many public rights of way in the New Forest which are shown on the maps.

THREE
The West Country

Hic jacet Arthurus, rex quondam, rex futurus
(Here lies Arthur, the once and future king)

The inscription on the tombstone of King Arthur
at Glastonbury, as recorded in the fifteenth
century *Red Book of Bath*

The West Country is one of my favourite regions, with the rolling plains of Wiltshire, the immense Bronze Age monuments at Stonehenge and Avebury, the vales of Dorset—Hardy's Wessex, the moors of Devon and the fantastic coast of Cornwall: a strip of granite jutting out into the ocean where no place is more than fifteen miles from the sea. There is the legend of Arthur and Camelot and the Round Table: druidical mystery and archaeological fact; and there are cream teas made from the amazing clotted cream that the South Devon cows have a penchant for making. You can try the Somerset and Devon cider, called locally "scrumpy", which is more bitter than the Kentish; and there is the Cornish pasty, a pastry-covered cake of mutton and potato, originally made as the tin miner's lunch and so durable is it that it could be dropped down a mine shaft and still come out whole!

There are three bike tours in the West Country, three long distance hiking paths and two shorter walks on the moors. A warning: Devon and Cornwall are not only popular with me: there are thousands of tourists in the high season. The main roads, in Cornwall especially, are one big caravan park in summer; so, if possible, try to visit the West Country either early or late in the season.

The bike routes in the West Country are covered by maps 15 and 16 in the Ordnance Survey Quarter-Inch Series, and by maps, 1, 2, 3, 4, 5, 7 and 8 in the Bartholomew 1:100,000 Series.

BIKING

SOMERSET and WILTSHIRE
(160 miles)

This is a tour of Arthurian and standing stone sites. In some ways it is an archaeological tour, because we will look at Stonehenge and potential candidates for "Camelot" by the evidence of the spade; but this is also a magical tour including, for example, the pagan mysteries of Avebury, Stonehenge and White Horse Hill, as well as cathedrals. The Arthurian legend is imbued with magic and mystery—the magic of the poet William Blake's *Albion,* the quest for the grail and the "second coming" of Arthur. Also it was on the plains of Wiltshire many millenia ago, that civilization began in the British Isles, when first Neolithic and then Bronze Age peoples settled here.

Salisbury to Hungerford (40 miles)

The lovely cathedral at Salisbury (LH) is unique in Britain as being the only cathedral completed from a single design and not added to continually over the centuries; it was begun in 1220 and finished sixty years later. Though it is unpleasant to be charged admission to a house of worship, do not be put off because you have to pay to get in: cathedrals are very expensive to maintain.

Two miles north of Salisbury on the small Woodford road, is Old Sarum, which was the cathedral city before the see was moved to New Sarum (Salisbury) in 1217. What you see today at Old Sarum are the remains of a Norman town with a cathedral and castle; but underlying that are the earthworks of an Iron Age fort. This is a long established site and it is said by some that Old Sarum was and is a natural holy place—a place where the conditions, whether magnetic or spiritual, are "right"—that Old Sarum is only one of a chain of natural holy places. John Michell, in his book, *View Over Atlantis,* talks of these holy hills and calls them "dragon hills". He describes them as part of a network of what the Chinese call the "dragon current"; this "current" has been variously interpreted as magnetic, gravitational and electrical waves. Interestingly enough, there are, all over England, a system of straight tracks, or leys, that seem to connect one holy site with another in unbelievably straight lines, as if laid out by someone who had a celestial vantage point. These "straight tracks" are very ancient; many have been incorporated into the Roman roads and though the Romans got the credit for the straightness, perhaps in reality, they were merely following much older trackways.

Sometimes the "holy" place is a church, sometimes standing stones. Christian churches were often built over older, pagan sites which might lead one to believe that certain places have a particular spiritual significance. Supposedly, the "ancients", whoever they were, knew how to control the so called "dragon current" and use it for their own purposes. The theorists say that we are sitting in the midst of a great natural cathedral and energy factory, but that it is just too large for us to see and we have lost the code. Hard-line archaeologists counter the theory by saying that the straight tracks were laid out as the shortest distance between two hills where sightings were taken, and that they were used by early settlers and merchants; as to the churches being built over older pagan sites, this was done primarily from a political motive: the early Christians wanted to completely supplant the older pagan forms, and what better way than to incorporate the old building in the new; and indeed this was an avowed practice of the early church. (There is an old trackway from Old Sarum to Stonehenge for those who want to walk.)

Continue north from Old Sarum through Woodford and turn left, west, on to the busy A303 for four miles to Stonehenge. This is probably the most famous prehistoric monument in Britain. It is not the work of the Druids, who, because they used it for their own purposes much later, have long been connected with the site; the Druids did not appear in Britain until the third century BC. In fact, archaeology has shown that Stonehenge was built and extended by different peoples over a period of about nine centuries between 2200 and 1300 BC. The earliest structures belong to the late Stone Age, but Stonehenge took its final shape during the Bronze Age. Some artifacts found at Stonehenge came originally from the Mycenaean and Minoan civilizations and point to trade links between the Mediterranean and the Bronze Age inhabitants of Britain in ancient times. When you see the size of the stones at Stonehenge you can get some idea of the extraordinary achievements of ancient technology and social organization. The smaller stones, known as *Bluestones* were transported from as far away as Wales. It has been suggested that Stonehenge was built primarily as a Solar temple, and it has long been known that the Axis of Stonehenge points to the midsummer sunrise; more recently, theorists have claimed that Stonehenge can be used as an

Somerset, Wiltshire and Dorset

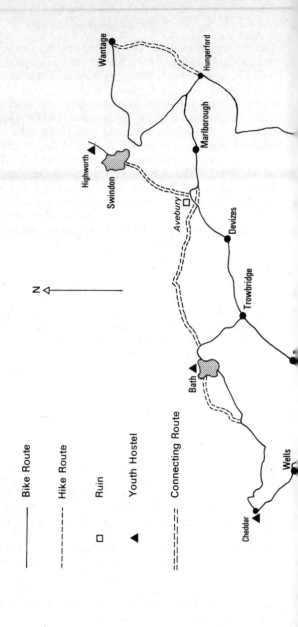

N ◁

——— Bike Route

- - - - - Hike Route

□ Ruin

▲ Youth Hostel

= = = = = Connecting Route

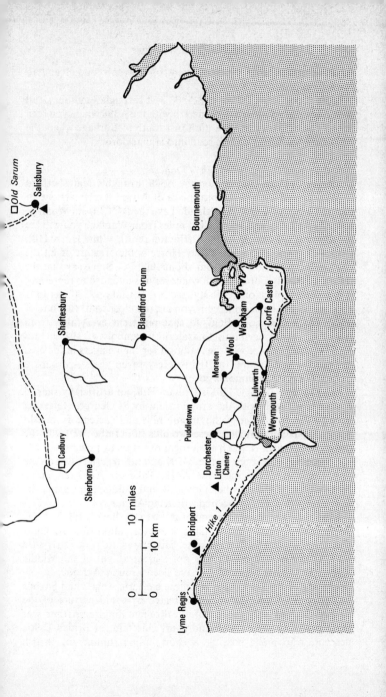

accurate predictor of the movement of heavenly bodies and to foretell eclipses.

From Stonehenge follow the A303 east through Amesbury and continue until you reach the junction with the A338 where you turn left to go north on the A338 until just south of Burbage where the A338 turns east; stay on this road into Hungerford.

Hungerford to Marlborough (45 miles)

From Hungerford continue on the A338 through Great Shefford to Wantage which was the birthplace of Alfred the Great, one of the first kings of a united England. Take the B4507 from Wantage towards Ashbury and about eight miles from Wantage you will see on your left (just opposite the Uffington road), White Horse Hill. I think that the Uffington White Horse is the greatest of all the chalk hill figures. It dates from about 1000 BC. Some say that the figure is actually a dragon, but whatever it is intended to represent, it is a superb piece of Celtic stylized art. It is about 360 feet long and can hardly be deciphered if you are too close to it. It is one of many chalk figures in England that represent everything from Iron Age fertility symbols to fraternity symbols of 1922. Until fairly recent times, it was the tradition for the villagers in the area to trim the sod around the figure every seven years—perhaps a magical number as numbers go.

Next to White Horse Hill is Dragon Hill, an artificially shaped mound associated with the dragon slain by St George. Referring back to the discussion of the dragon hills and currents from Old Sarum, you could say that these two hills fit in rather well with the theory of magic hills which are a focus of magnetic powers.

Proceed into Ashbury on the B4507 and through the town on the same road until you meet the A419. Take the A419 left going south-east to Badbury where you will find Liddington Castle, the first site on this tour associated with King Arthur.

Medieval and even contemporary writers have exploited the Arthurian story so much that it is almost impossible to know where reality and fiction separate. Historians are now fairly sure that Arthur existed but he was not a great knight of the Middle Ages. He is now believed to have lived around AD 500, at the beginning of the Dark Ages when the barbaric Angles and Saxons began pouring into the vacuum created by the departure of the Roman legions and decline of the Roman Empire. Arthur was most probably some rough-and-ready chieftain, of British/Celtic descent, who made possible a short indian summer of British culture before the barbarians overran the island.

It is thought that Arthur commanded a group of warriors, who perhaps fought from horseback, something that the Saxons had never before experienced; and that he was successful in repulsing the barbaric advance for at least a generation. Arthur's importance to history is as a wise field general: by temporarily stopping the advance of the Saxons he gave European civilization a second chance. And this is not an over-statement: the generation of peace that followed Arthur's stand against the barbarian invasions gave the monasteries in England and Ireland a chance to flourish; and it was these monasteries more than any other one institution that were responsible for the preservation of Western learning through the long and bleak Dark Ages that ensued.

Ireland, especially, became a seat of learning for all Europe during the next centuries (as you will discover if you follow the tours of Ireland). The Angles and Saxons did eventually conquer the island, but they were not the same people whom Arthur had defeated a generation before. They were more settled and had become more civilized, due partly to the Christian missionaries at work among them, and so were more willing to live in accord with their former enemies. The historic "Camelot" was, in fact, this brief Celtic rebirth in the early sixth century—not the Hollywood fairyland of courtly love and jousts.

Liddington Castle is just a nine hundred foot hill, but it may have been the site of the historic battle of Mount Badon, fought in AD 520, in which Arthur defeated the invaders and gave Britain a breathing space.

Continue on the A419 towards Hungerford again, but take the Ramsbury (L) turning to the left, west, before Hungerford and continue on through Ramsbury to Marlborough (L).

Marlborough to Wells (50 miles)

From Marlborough, take the A4 for about seven miles and turn right, to the north-west, at West Kennet for Avebury, a couple of miles up the road.

The Avebury site is much bigger than Stonehenge—the stones around the village are not just random boulders, but the remains of an immense stone circle. The ditch and embankment around the stones are about a mile in circumference. Interestingly enough, the ditch is inside the bank at Avebury; normally, when there is a ditch and bank construction, the ditch is outside the bank as a kind of fortification, giving the defenders an advantage over the attackers as they scrambled into the ditch and up the wall of the embankment. But at Avebury, it is as if the embankment and ditch were designed to keep someone or something inside the circle, rather than out. The stone circle at Avebury probably had the same function as Stonehenge, but so many stones are missing that there is no evidence that it was a seasonal clock.

An avenue of standing stones called the Kennet Avenue, leads from Avebury to a sanctuary on Overton Hill. Silbury Hill is also close by. It is thought that this huge, artificial hill was originally part of the Avebury complex, though even older, dating from perhaps 2000 BC. This is one of the largest man-made mounds in the world and its purpose is still unknown. There is a museum near Avebury church and the beginnings of an excellent long distance path, the Ridgeway Path, not far away (see under *Hiking*); there is a place next to the car park to leave bikes if you decide to walk to any of the Ridgeway.

Take the A361 south to Devizes (LC), where there is an important collection of Bronze Age urns, beakers and other grave ware excavated from long barrows on Salisbury Plain in the nineteenth century. It is located on Long Street, and open Tuesdays to Saturdays, eleven a.m. to five p.m.

From Devizes, take the A361 south-west through Trowbridge and Frome (L) to Shepton Mallet where you take the A371 into Wells (LC).

There is a good optional route of about forty-five miles that you may wish to make from Trowbridge via Bath and back to Wells. Take the A363 north from Trowbridge through Bradford-on-Avon (L) to the intersection with the A4 where you turn left for Bath (LCH), only a few miles away. This route is fairly hilly, but worth it. Bath is a lovely city—founded originally by the Romans as a natural spa; with its lovely crescents, it is a showcase of Georgian architecture.

Take the A367 south from Bath for several miles until you come to the B3115, turn off to the right, south-west, for Timsbury. Continue through Timsbury on the B3115 till it meets the A39 where you turn left, south-west through Chewton Mendip. After Chewton Mendip you will come to the junction with the B3135. Turn right on to this road to go over the Mendip Hills to Cheddar (LCH) and the magnificent Cheddar Gorge (the inspiration of the hymn *Rock of Ages Cleft for Me*).

From Cheddar travel south-east on the A371 to Wells. The cathedral at Wells dominates the town; it is early English Gothic built in the twelfth century and looks every inch the home of a bishop. There is superb medieval sculpture on the front, and amazingly modern-looking back-to-back arches surrounding the altar; they look like something by Frank Lloyd Wright, but are of course, twelfth century.

Wells to South Cadbury (25 miles)

Take the A39 south into Glastonbury (L) or Street (H), only a few miles away. Glastonbury is reputed to be Avalon, the burial place of King Arthur (who, according to legend, is not dead but sleeping in a cave waiting to return). Edward I, in an attempt to subdue the Welsh by putting to rest once and for all their legend that Arthur would come again, dug up the reputed coffin of Arthur at Glastonbury, removed the bones and put them on show; however the bones did not put the legend to rest; for some, Arthur will always be the once and future king. Not only is Glastonbury the burial place of Arthur, it was also the home of the first and most powerful abbey in England, founded in the seventh century, a place where Britons and Saxons worshipped and lived in supposed harmony—a considerable achievement in those troubled days. You can see the ruins of the old abbey, the Lady Chapel and the refectory with its fireplace in every corner. Glastonbury is also associated with the mystery of the Holy Grail. Legend tells how Joseph of Arimathea came to Glastonbury with the chalice which was used in the Last Supper and which contained drops of Christ's blood. The legend of the chalice, or grail, became incorporated into the stories of King Arthur and his Knights of the Round Table.

Overlooking Glastonbury is the Tor—an eerie, cone-shaped hill that looks man-made but is supposedly natural. At the top of the Tor are the remains of the medieval chapel of St Michael. This hill was thought to be a Dark Age habitation of some sort, but whether a fortress or a shrine is not known; it could have served as part of a beacon alarm system, high as it is over the flat Somerset plain. There are the remains of a complicated terracing system on the slopes, said by some to be a magical maze used in a religious initiation ceremony. Others say that the terracing is only the result of natural erosion; but the mystery remains and the digging goes on when money is available.

It is not far from Glastonbury to Arthur's "Camelot". Continue south through Street and take the B3151 through Somerton, a lovely, stone-built market town, towards Ilchester.

About a mile north of Ilchester, you turn left on to the A303 going north-east through Sparkford. Two miles beyond Sparkford there is a minor road to the right, south, to South Cadbury, where, not far from the village, you will find the hill of Cadbury Castle, reputed to be Camelot.

There have been many candidates for the court of Arthur, but the legend has long been that it was situated at Cadbury Castle. Archaeological digs in the last few years have gone a long way towards verifying tradition. But there is no mighty, medieval castle; all that remains of Arthur's castle is an embankment system; and little remains of the houses but post-holes. The earthworks were originally Iron Age fortifications, but were obviously rebuilt in the sixth century. The re-building was quite novel for its day and the structure could easily have been the residence of some Dark Age chieftain such as Arthur might have been. The excavations have shown that this Dark Age chieftain was more Celtic than Arthur was thought to have been, for the fortifications show little Roman influence.

From the top of Cadbury you can see an impressive view of Glastonbury Tor in the distance.

THOMAS HARDY'S DORSET
(100 miles)

This tour visits many of the sites described in the novels of Thomas Hardy. If you are joining this tour from the last one, follow the South Cadbury road farther south till it joins the B3145 going south into Sherbourne (L), which is a pleasant country town with an abbey, and a castle built by Sir Walter Raleigh. Sherbourne is Sherton Abbas in *Tess of the d'Urbervilles*.

Sherbourne to Puddletown (45 miles)

Continue east out of Sherbourne on the A30. After about ten miles, turn right, south, on to the B3092 and go through the village of Marnhull, the village where Tess grew up, called Marlott in the novel. Continue south on the same road to Sturminster Newton and then north-east on the B309 to Shaftesbury (L), which is *Shaston* (the ancient name of Shaftesbury) in *Jude the Obscure*. This is the place where Sue Bridehead jumped from the third storey window.

Continue south from Shaftesbury on the A350 to Blandford

Forum (L), Shotsford Forum in *Far From the Madding Crowd*: this is a Georgian town set on the banks of the river Stour. The town hall and the Church of St Peter and St Paul are lovely buildings. Take the A354 south-west out of Blandford for four or five miles to the Milton Abbas turning to the right. Follow this road into Milton Abbas, a pretty little thatched village built in the seventeenth century by the Earl of Dorchester. The Earl had had the earlier market town here destroyed because it spoiled his view. This is the setting of Middleton Abbey in Hardy's tale, *The Woodlanders*. Continue through the village on the same road until you rejoin the A354 where you turn left, going south-west into Puddleton, Weatherbury in *Far from the Madding Crowd*. Waterston Manor just west of the town, is the site of Bathsheba's house in the same novel.

Puddletown to Dorchester (55 miles)

Go east out of Puddletown on the A35 to Bere Regis, Kingsbere in *Tess of the d'Urbervilles*. Stay on the A35 east after Bere Regis for about two miles until a turning on to a minor road to the right, south-east, for Wareham (LC), about five miles away; this is Anglebury in *Return of the Native*. Near Wareham is Cloud's Hill, the lonely moorland cottage which T. E. Lawrence (Lawrence of Arabia) rented after 1923. From Wareham take the A351 south-east to Corfe Castle, a picturebook castle and village. The castle was built in 1280 by Edward I, and is Coversgage Castle in Hardy's tale, *The Hand of Ethelberta*. Take a minor road west to the B3070 and turn left, south, to Lulworth Cove, a wide, three mile long bay with good swimming and many tourists; there is also good fossil hunting here. Nearby is Durdle Dor, a natural limestone arch jutting out into the sea. This figures in a scene in *Far From the Madding Crowd*. On your way to Lulworth you will go through East Lulworth; the castle there is the archetypal castle, but it was actually built in the seventeenth century as a second home by a local lord.

Leave Lulworth by the B3071 going north to Wool (L), which is Wellbridge in *Tess of the d'Urbervilles*, where Tess and her husband Angel go for their honeymoon. From Wool go north on a minor road to Moreton in the Blackmore Vale, where Tess goes after her disgrace and where she first meets her future husband, Angel Clare. Continuing along this minor road, you will reach the B3390 where you turn left, travelling south-west, to meet the A352 where you turn right, west, to Broadmayne, and then left, going west, on a minor road to the A354. Turn right, north, on this road, to Dorchester.

About two miles south of Dorchester, you will pass Maiden Castle which figures in a scene from *The Mayor of Casterbridge*. Maiden Castle is a complex system of earth ramparts and ditches, the best example of an Iron Age fort in England. A skeleton was found here with a catapult bolt in its spine, providing dramatic evidence for archaeologists of the Roman siege of AD 43.

Stay on the A354 into Dorchester (LC), the setting of Casterbridge in *The Mayor of Casterbridge*. This is an historic town, where there has been a settlement since 500 BC in the Iron Age. There is a good county museum containing a reconstruction of Thomas Hardy's study as well as finds from Maiden Castle.

DEVON and CORNWALL
(370 miles)

This is a long tour that starts in South Devon at Exeter and traverses Dartmoor, entering Cornwall and travelling up the west coast back into North Devon, across Exmoor, through Minehead on the coast, to end up in Bridgwater for connections to the next touring area to the North. The route passes through some of the best scenery in England, from the dramatic heights of the moors, to the grandeur of the Cornish Riviera. It is a hilly ride, difficult in some places, and could take up to two weeks to complete, depending on your biking speed. Do not hesitate to break it into smaller tours.

Devon and Cornwall both take their names from the Celtic. Cornwall's ancient name was *Dod-nys* (Totnes is the name of a present day town) which means the "projecting island". In the tenth century, however, the name *Cornweles* appears, signifying in Welsh the "Horn of Britain". Devon comes from the Celtic *Dyfnamt,* meaning "dark and deep valleys".

One word of caution before you start the tour: Cornwall is the end of the line for trains and there are large areas not serviced by the railway. There are routes down to Penzance in the south, but none on the west coast itself. Inland there are stations at Barnstaple in the north and Bodmin in the centre near the coastal town of Padstow.

Exeter to Truro (58 miles)
Exeter (L) is Devon's county town. There is a castle which was

built by William the Conqueror, an excellent cathedral where you can see the world's longest expanse of Gothic vaulting; there are also some good brasses. From Exeter travel south-west on the B3212 through Dunsford (H) and Moretonhampstead, a pleasant little village, and on to Dartmoor.

Dartmoor is a national park. It covers an area of 365 square miles. The core of the park consists of two main upland plateaux separated at Two Bridges by 'B' class roads. The northern moor is the larger of the two and rises to 2083 feet at High Willhays. But be careful in this part, for there is a military firing range extending from Okehampton as far as Two Bridges. These two plateaux are wilderness areas of bog and cotton-grass; to the east, the land is more arable. Granite outcroppings called tors jut out of the landscape, as do prehistoric stone monuments. Medieval trackways such as the Abbot's Way, the Jobber's Way and the Lich Way link many of the medieval settlements on the moor (see under *Hiking*). The moor is a bleak and wonderful place and the land is open: a great place to wander in. Watch out for the buzzards with their wild, ringing, mewing call; a buzzard looks like a small eagle with a wing-span of about four feet. There are also ravens with their deep-throated croak, which lends bleakness and mystery to the moor. Cattle, sheep and wild ponies graze on the moor. Beyond Moretonhampstead there are many minor roads which go into the heart of the moor. You may like to take a minor road south to Widecomb-in-the-Moor and Bucklands-in-the-Moor, both lovely, and very typical of moorland villages. There are also many tors to be seen on the route.

Continue on the B3212 to Two Bridges where there is a National Park Office which has many leaflets describing walks and excursions on the moor; Dartmoor is also good horse-riding country and information about this can be found at the office.

Take the A384 west to Tavistock (HCL) where Sir Francis Drake was born. This was rich copper mining country in the nineteenth century. From Tavistock take the A390 south-west through Liskeard to where the road forks, then take the A38, to the right, for Bodmin (CL).

There is also an alternative route from Tavistock to Bodmin, for those who really like the moor. Take the A384 north from Launceston, where there is a Norman castle and the church of St Mary Magdalene. From there join the A30 across Bodmin Moor to the south. This route crosses twelve miles of open moorland, with cattle and ponies and many tors, and takes you into Bodmin, a

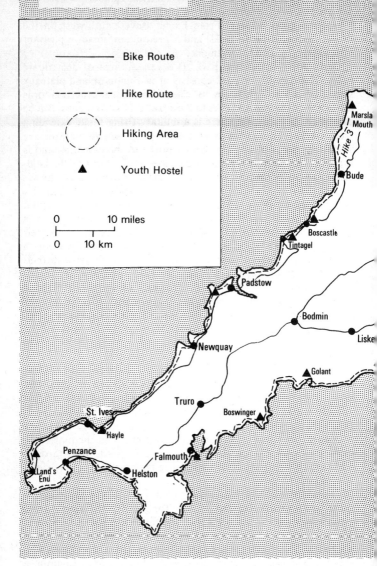

Devon and Cornwall

——————	Bike Route
– – – – –	Hike Route
◯	Hiking Area
▲	Youth Hostel

0   10 miles

0   10 km

Marsla Mouth

Hike 3

Bude

Boscastle

Tintagel

Padstow

Bodmin

Liske

Newquay

Golant

Truro

Boswinger

St. Ives

Hayle

Penzance

Falmouth

Land's End

Helston

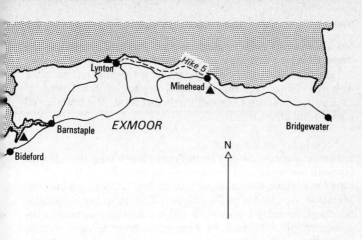

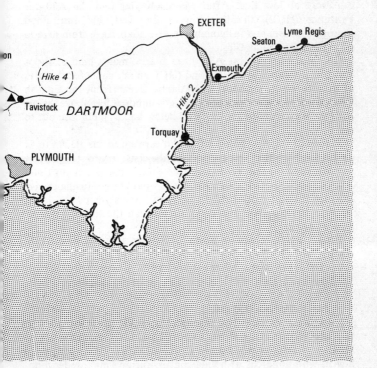

town with roots back in the Iron Age. The moor surrounds the town, giving it a deep sense of Celtic mystery.

Take the A30 south from Bodmin, till it branches left on to the A39 for Truro (L), the unofficial capital of the Duchy of Cornwall, containing Cornwall's only cathedral. The town is well planned and pleasant.

Truro to St Ives (62 miles)

Continue south on the A39 from Truro till you meet the A394 for Helston; go through Helston and stay on the A394 for Marazion, a little town whose name means "market jew". Out to sea opposite Marazion lies St Michael's Mount. This is a hotch-potch of buildings, formerly a monastery, and nowhere near as lovely as its namesake off the coast of France; however it does provide impressive views of the mainland to which it is connected by a causeway at low tide. After Marazion you join the A30 for Penzance (HCL), the Brighton of the west, but fun; good Victorian houses in a fashionable resort. Boats leave from here to go to the balmy Scilly Isles.

Continue south on the A30 through a no-man's land of shops and petrol stations to Land's End (HC): an apt name for the strip of granite which separates the Atlantic Ocean from the English Channel. It is a bare stone plateau eight-hundred feet above the sea with the waves pounding the cliffs below and a lighthouse out to sea.

Return to the A30 going north and turn on to the B3305 to St Just (CL). Now that you are back on the coast, try to stay as close as possible to the sea. To do this necessitates changing many times from one minor road to another and it would be confusing to give instructions and road numbers here, so just use maps and logic, stick to the coastline and continue through the towns I will be describing.

From St Just continue north to St Ives (CL), a nineteenth-century artists' colony which still has a bit of that air lingering even today in spite of the tourists; it is renowned for its Mediterranean light, and that is not a type of draught beer!

St Ives to Padstow (55 miles)

Go north-east from St Ives through Hayle (HCL), Portreath (C), St Agnes (C), and then to Newquay (CL) which is about the largest holiday resort you will find in Cornwall. There is a good, open beach, with hundreds of holidaymakers turning pink under a hot summer sun. From Newquay follow the coastline to Padstow (HCL) which is an attractive, fairly unspoilt small medieval town.

Padstow to Hartland (61 miles)

Take the ferry from Padstow across the inlet to Rock and from there to St Minerva and Port Isaac, a fishing village full of slate houses, and on up the coast through Delabole to Tintagel (HCL). The Norman castle at Tintagel juts out into the ocean and has almost been cut off from the mainland by the action of the sea. This is the legendary birthplace of King Arthur, and there have been archaeological finds which indicate that there were buildings here at the time of King Arthur. Tintagel itself is a pleasant little town—its name tells you something about the former importance of the tin trade in Cornwall: the Phoenicians used to sail all the way to England for tin. See the old Post Office in town and have a cream tea at one of the tea houses.

Continue north from Tintagel to Boscastle (H), a tiny village built on the hillside around a tiny harbour. Visit the museum of witchcraft and sorcery, one of the best of its kind in Europe: there is everything from the paintings of the diabolical Aleister Crowley to the thigh bone of a Tibetan sorcerer-priest. From Boscastle, go north away from the coast, through Poundstock and back to the coast at Bude (CL), a modern resort where you can surf. From Bude take the A39 into Devon at Hartland (H).

Hartland to Exford (50 miles)

Stay on the A39 from Hartland into Bideford (CL) with its medieval streets, then on through Instow (H) to Barnstaple (C), where there is an interesting museum in the Guildhall containing a collection of plate and ancient seals. From Barnstaple take a minor road north-east to Brayford, and from Brayford take another minor road north-east to Simonsbath in Exmoor.

Exmoor is a national park though smaller than Dartmoor and accentuated more by its deep-cut gulleys, called combes, than by tors; it is bare and windswept on the heights which are covered with heather and grasses, yet there are wooded valleys rich in ferns. There are many prehistoric remains, such as stone circles. The name Exmoor derives from the Celtic word *isca*, meaning water, and refers to the river which flows across the moor. Dunkery Beacon, which stands at 1708 feet, is the highest point and catches all the weather from the Atlantic. There are about sixty inches of rainfall per year. The ancient Forest of Exmoor which lies around

Simonsbath was once the preserve of kings, and like the New Forest is not necessarily wooded. There are ponies and buzzards, as on Dartmoor, but not so much open moorland on which to ramble. The Oare Valley to the north-east is the Doone Valley from R. D. Blackmore's *Lorna Doone.*

At Simonsbath you have the option of continuing across the moor to Exford (HC) on the main east route, the B3358, or going north along the coast to the twin resorts of Lynton and Lynmouth (HCL), both very pretty and green spots. If taking the coastal route, continue east from Lynton on the A39 through the town of Porlock, which was once on the sea, but is now a good mile inland. Stay on this route to Minehead (HCL).

Exford to Bridgport (50 miles)

From Exford there is a minor road going north over the moor to meet the coast road, the A39, just before Porlock. Turn right on the A39, going east through Porlock and into Minehead (HCL). Minehead is an old port and still maintains a village air despite the holiday camps which surround it like so many armies laying siege.

From Minehead, continue east on the A39 through Dunster with its castle and yarn market; Dunster is also thought to have been an early residence of Arthur before he moved to South Cadbury. Just east of Dunster take a minor road off the A39 to the left towards the coast to Watchet where Samuel Taylor Coleridge was inspired to write *The Ancient Mariner.* Go through the little town and continue on the minor road, east, back to the A39 at Willington. Stay on the A39 through Holford (H) and Nether Stowey, where Coleridge rented a cottage from 1797 to 1800 for the grand sum of seven pounds per annum and where he wrote *The Ancient Mariner* and *Kubla Kahn.* The cottage is near the west end of the town and can be visited.

Continue east to Bridgwater (CL) and the end of the tour. This town is on major routes and has a railway station.

HIKING

There is plenty of opportunity for weeks or days or just hours of walking in the West Country. There are over four hundred miles of long distance coastal path, from Studland, near Poole Harbour in

Dorset, all the way around Cornwall to Marsland Mouth just north of Bude. For convenience I have divided the South-West Peninsula Coast Path into three sections: Dorset, South Devon, and Cornwall. A useful publication describing the whole path, which can be bought at bookshops in the area of the hikes, is Edward C. Pyatt's *Coastal Paths of the Southwest.* Dartmoor, Exmoor and Bodmin Moor also offer splendid possibilities for long and short walks on open moorland.

NOTE: a section of the long Ridgeway Path passes through this area, and though most of it is included in the next chapter, the Heart of England, the section of the Ridgeway from White Horse Hill near Uffington, to near Avebury, coincides very well with part of a bike route included in this chapter; but I have not described any of the Ridgeway in this section, so those wanting to walk that path should see under *Hiking* in the following chapter.

THE DORSET COAST PATH
(72 miles)

This is a section from Studland in the east to Lyme Regis in the west. In most areas the path stays close to the coast and there is little difficulty in navigation; but there are places where the path meanders inland, and when there are significant changes in direction they are indicated by branded wooden signs bearing the words *Coast Path*. These signs are particularly in evidence where you could lose your way on a paved surface. The stylized acorn, symbol of the long distance paths, can be seen at points along the path as a waymarker, confirming the line of path. The route is covered by the following Ordnance Survey Maps in the 1:50,000 Series: 193, Taunton to Lyme Regis; 194, Dorchester and Weymouth; and 195, Bournemouth and Purbeck. The maps show rights of way along the path and by using them it will be possible to find feeder routes on to and off the path, should you want to make a detour to find lodgings along the way. This path is within the capabilities of any fairly fit person: there are no very great climbs, but watch out near the cliffs, especially if mists start rolling in, or after rain when footholds might be slippery. When planning the day's walk on this terrain, it is always sensible to allow extra time for changes in direction and altitude. There is one place in particular where the hikers should be careful and that is the firing range between Kimmeridge and Lulworth Cove.

1. Studland to Lyme Regis (72 miles)

You can start this path a little east of Studland, or at Poole or Bournemouth where you can catch a bus to Sandbanks. From Sandbanks you take the regular ferry services across Poole Harbour to South Haven Point, where you can begin walking along the edge of the dunes above the sandy beach to Studland.

The path from Studland climbs up to Handfast Point above Old Harry Rocks and the Pinnacle, and continues over the end of the chalk hill range at Ballard Down, descending from there into Swanage (HLC). This section of the path is on the spit of land known as the Isle of Purbeck. From Swanage the coast goes south, and you follow it along cliffs formed of Purbeck stone past Durlston Head, through the abandoned quarry known as Tilly Whim Caves, along Dancing Ledge and Seacombe Cliff, behind Winspit to the tiny Norman church, still in use, which surmounts the limestone headland of St Aldhelm's Head. From here there are views of the Isle of Wight to the east and of Portland to the west. The path descends through the landslip of Chapman's Pool and along the shale cliffs, passing above Kimmeridge Ledges and into the village of Kimmeridge.

The route from Kimmeridge to Lulworth Cove (L) necessitates a detour because of the firing ranges. This detour is necessary on most weekdays, but firing is not usual on Fridays and weekends, and it is then sometimes possible to avoid this detour by walking a mile to the north to Steeple, from there to Whiteway Hill and then on the road over the ranges to East Lulworth and into Lulworth Cove, where you return to the coast path. *But always check to make sure before setting off across the firing ranges:* telephone the range officer at Bindon Abbey, or look for announcements in the local paper.

The detour which avoids the firing range is eighteen miles long, going by minor roads and path to Corfe Castle, and from there by local bus services to Wareham and Wool. Then you can walk the five miles from Wool on the B3071 road to Lulworth Cove. Continue west from Lulworth Cove along the coast path past Durdle Dor, then up and over the five hundred foot cliff at White Northe and along the coast below the site of Ringstead village to Osmington Mills (C).

At this point the coastal path divides giving you an inland alternative. The inland route goes north-east close by the enormous chalk equestrian figure cut into the hillside near Sutton Poyntz, and through Bincombe up to the Hardy Monument, at eight-hundred feet, from which there are some good views. After the Hardy Monument you may have to leave the path because of right of way difficulties. For this detour, take the road southwest all the way to White Hill and from there continue on the path along the ridge of the White Hill via Abbotsbury Castle and Limekiln Hill to West Bexington.

The coast route from Osmington Mills continues along the cliffs to Overcombe and into Weymouth (LC), which is a large seaside resort with an elegant promenade of Georgian and Victorian homes. Beyond Weymouth, the path resumes at the ruins of Sandsfoot Castle in Portland Harbour. It continues south for a while, then turns west to Langton Herring where it leaves the coast.

The section of path between Bridge Lane (Ordnance Survey map reference point 605829), and Horsepool Farm (579846) should be by-passed by turning north-west on to a footpath at Bridge Lane to New Barn (598834). From New Barn continue north-west along the New Barn road via Walls Down to Horsepool Farm where the path may be re-joined going north-west to Abbotsbury (L) with its ancient Swannery built by the Benedictines and still housing hundreds of swans. After Abbotsbury the path returns to the coast at Chesil Beach, following the beach into West Bexington where it joins the inland alternative route.

From West Bexington the path continues behind Chesil Beach to Burton Bradstock, and from there through West Bay, Eype Mouth, Seatown and then climbs up to the highest point on the south coast at Golden Cap. Descend from here to the footbridge over the River Char and back down to sea-level at Charmouth. From Charmouth the path goes by the golf course and to the eastern boundary of Lyme Regis (L), opposite the cemetery gates. Lyme Regis was once a port and is now sheltered by an ancient, curved breakwater called the Cobb. Lyme got its royal name during the reign of Edward I, whose name crops up all over the West Country. Both Lyme Regis and Charmouth are a fossil hunter's paradise: ammonites up to two feet in length and the teeth or vertebrae of marine reptiles can sometimes be found. Beyond Lyme Regis, the path leads west to the Devon boundary where the next section of the coast path, the South Devon Coast Path, begins.

THE SOUTH DEVON COAST PATH
(93 miles)

This is relatively easy walking through one of the busier coastal areas. The path passes through many bustling seaside resorts but also offers long stretches of unspoilt scenery. It starts on the Devon boundary near Lyme Regis in the east and ends at Turnchapel near Plymouth in the west. Along the route there are limestone cliffs, river estuaries, mica schist cliffs and limestone promontories. Of the resorts, Beer and Brixham are probably the nicest, i.e. less spoilt and day-trippy than others such as Torquay and Paignton, through which the coast path does not even take you; in fact, the official pamphlet describing the path leaves it to each individual to find "his way through the built-up areas of Paignton and Torquay."

The maps for this path are the Ordnance Survey 1:50,000 Series: 201, Plymouth to Launceston; 202, Torbay and South Dartmoor; 192, Exeter and Sidmouth; and 193, Taunton and Lyme Regis. The way is marked with the acorn symbol. When the path diverges greatly from the coastline, it is marked by oak signs bearing the words *Coastal Path,* plus the acorn. As always, be careful along the cliffs, especially if mists come in from the sea. Otherwise, this path is not a difficult one and is suitable for anyone who is reasonably fit; it is not an endurance test. Accommodation can be found in most towns and villages and at hostels along the route.

2. *Lyme Regis to Turnchapel (93 miles)*

The path begins just west of Lyme Regis at the Devon boundary and follows the coastal landslip west, climbing up to the golf links near Seaton and then into the town. Seaton is like many of the resorts you will pass through on this walk; small, with a pebble beach which will be full or empty of people, depending upon the time of year.

From Seaton continue along the coast to Beer (LH), a cosy little resort which you may be able to reach on your first night. From Beer continue west through Branscombe into Sidmouth (L) which still has tinges of Elegance and Gentility left over from the days when Queen Victoria stayed there.

You will have to go inland from Sidmouth to cross the River Otter by a footbridge, then come back on to the coast on the other side of Budleigh Salterton and continue along the coast to Straight Point. Here the path again diverges from the line of the coast, going behind the ranges, and then on into Exmouth (L), a large, popular resort. Take the ferry across the Exe from Exmouth to Starcross where you take the road south-east to Dawlish Warren station. Then take a footpath west and just inland from the railway to Dawlish, another seaside resort. From there proceed on the path into Teignmouth, cross the River Teign, then continue south-west to Hope's Nose through Babbacombe.

At Hope's Nose the coastal path stops for a short distance. You are just north of the resort of Torquay, but unless you want to spend some time in "England's Cannes", I advise you to take a bus from Torquay through Paignton to the Churston Golf Course overlooking Tor Bay, where you can regain the coast path. The path here skirts the golf course and continues in a curve south-east to Brixham (L) which has a lovely, old harbour with a replica of Drake's *Golden Hind*. On the far side of Brixham the path continues south-west past the limestone promontory of Berry Head, following the coast closely to Coleton.

At Man Sands (Ordnance Survey map reference point 922534), going towards Kingswear, there is difficulty with right of way. From Man Sands follow a country lane to Woodhuish (913528) and continue in a south-westerly direction; the country lane turns into a path which runs south-west into Mill Bay Cove, (892504) just south-east of Kingswear.

From Kingswear cross the River Dart to Dartmouth by ferry. The path follows the coast from Dartmouth Castle to Warren Point where it goes a bit inland to Stoke Fleming and Strete. Take the old coach road down the hill to Strete Gate and then follow the narrow ridge of land between the Ley and the Sea to Slapton Ley, continuing south-west to Torcross and climbing up to Start Point (H). From here follow the clifftop to Prawle Point and Gara Rock, which is excellent open cliff walking owned by the National Trust. The path descends to the ferry crossing at Salcombe Harbour (H). Take the ferry across the harbour and continue in a generally north-westerly direction along the coast into another National Trust area of cliffs which stretch from Sharpitor, near Salcombe, through Bolt Head and Bolt Tail to Hope Cove and Thurlestone Sands. Continue north-west to Bantham where you take the ferry across the Avon and thence into Bigbury-on-Sea (H).

Follow the cliffs from Bigbury until you come to the mouth of the River Erme. It may be possible to cross the estuary by wading at low tide, or by fording the river about a mile upstream; if not, you will have to go a further two miles inland to use the road crossing. Whichever you do, make your way from the other side of the river to Mothecombe on the coast. From here continue along the coast north-west to the estuary of the River Yealm which you cross by ferry to Wembury Bay, and then continue west from there to Wembury Point where you come back out on to the cliffs. Proceed north-west via Heybrook Bay and Bovisand Bay to near Stamford Fort, which the path skirts on the west side. Continue into Turnchapel which is north-east of Plymouth Sound. There are transport connections and a hostel in Plymouth, which is a big city with an interesting history. Unfortunately it was bombed heavily in the war and the rebuilding is not all that admirable.

This is the end of the route: to the west of Plymouth is the Cornwall Coast Path.

THE CORNWALL COAST PATH
(268 miles)

For me, this is the best of all the coastal paths for scenery and walking, its closest competitor being the wild and difficult Pembrokeshire Coast Path in South Wales. The Cornwall path stretches from near Plymouth, in the south-east, to the boundary with Devon in the north at Marsland Mouth. Along its route you will find peace and relaxation away from the busy lanes of Cornwall, while still being able to enjoy that particular aura and dramatic feeling that the coast of Cornwall provides.

This path is a huge undertaking, so do not feel compelled to walk the whole way: pick and choose the stretches which are the best or most convenient for you. My favourite part of the path is the west stretch between Boscastle and Land's End, where the cliff scenery is especially good and where there are several hostels to break your journey into comfortable day-walks. Refer to the bike route in this chapter—which covers most of the same ground—for descriptions of places and for lodgings. The part of the path between Bude and Boscastle is perhaps the only difficult stretch, because it is so uninhabited.

In the Ordnance Survey 1:50,000 Series, carry: 190, Bude; 200, Newquay; 203, Land's End; 204, Truro; 201, Plymouth to Launceston. There is also an official handbook published by the Cornwall Tourist Board, called the *Cornwall Coast Path* which has a good map in it plus an accommodation guide list; and there are several other books about the Cornwall path, which you can buy when you are in the area.

This path took a long time to plan. It incorporates many old coastguard paths as well as many new ones. Stay close to the sea and you will be able to find the path with ease; when the path deviates inland, the way is marked by oak signs bearing the words *Coast Path* and the acorn symbol. Be sure to allow plenty of extra time when planning itineraries for changes in direction and level; and watch out along the cliffs for mists, gusty winds and slippery rocks after rain.

3. *Plymouth to Marsland Mouth (268 miles)*

From Plymouth take the ferry to Cremyll on the Tamar estuary where the path begins. Walk along the seaward edge of Mount Edgcumbe Park, through the villages of Kingsand and Cawsand to Penlee Point. From here the path goes inland a bit to avoid the rifle ranges on Blarrick Cliff, and continues to Crafthole (L) on the coast and then to Rame Head and Whitsand Bay to Portwrinkle. At the time of writing, there was still a problem with the section between Portwrinkle, (Ordnance Survey map reference point 355539) and St Germans Beacon (334541) so use the coast road for this section.

Continue north-west through Downderry (L) to East and West Looe and along a lovely stretch by Portnalder Bay and Talland Bay to Polperro (L). From Downderry to Seaton the path runs along the foot of the cliffs just above the high water line and if there is an exceptionally high tide it is best to walk along the nearby coast road.

From Polperro, follow the cliffs west to Polruan where you take a ferry across the river Fowey to the town of Fowey. From here continue west along the cliffs past Gribbin Head to Polkeriss and north to Polmear where you must take the main road into the port of Par. From Par the path veers south through the tiny port of Charlestown, then on to St Austell Bay and Mevagissey. It continues south around Dodman Point and then west to Hemmick Beach, past the grounds of Caerhays Castle, and around Veryan Bay, Nay Head and St Anthony Head. At St Anthony in Roseland you take a ferry which runs regularly in the summer (or hire a private boat in other seasons to avoid the long inland detour) to St Mawes, and from there take another ferry to Falmouth (LH), a resort and dockyard situated on the estuary of seven rivers.

From Falmouth the path continues south-west to the Helford River which can be crossed by ferry. From the other side the path leads to Dennis Head and then south to Gillan Harbour which has no ferry service but can normally be waded at low tide. At other times walk along the road to St Anthony on the north side of the creek to the head of Gillan Creek and on to Carne, and from there into Flushing. You rejoin the coast at Porthallow, go inland again via Trenance, back out to the little harbour of Porthoustock and inland to Rosenithon, continuing near Manacle Point so as to avoid cliffside quarries north of the village of Coverack. There is a difficult section of coast between Coverack and Cadgwith. From Cadgwith you continue to Lizard Point, the most southerly place in England. This whole peninsula is spectacular with high cliffs and pounding surf.

After Lizard point you go north-west and pass Kynance Cove, where you can see the cliffs at their best, then up to Mullion Cove and into Porthleven (L). The path continues from here through Marazion and into Penzance at the Albert Pier, on the seaward side of the railway line. From Penzance (H), the path continues along the coast past some superb scenery at Mousehole and on out to Land's End (H).

After Land's End there is a long stretch of exceptionally fine and rugged coastline to St Ives and Carbis Bay to the River Hayle. In the absence of a ferry service, you have to walk into the town of Hayle (H), around the head of the estuary by road to Lelant and continue north to pick up the path again (at 549379). If there is a ferry running, it will take you across to Hayle Towans from where you can walk across sand dunes and cliffs to the dramatic high cliffs at Godrevy Point. From here continue north-east into Portreath and around St Agnes Head to Perranporth, a popular resort.

The route follows Perran Beach north-east from Perranporth then goes inland past the little church of St Piran, across the sands to Gear and then by road to the north end of Penhale Sands. From there, by way of Holywell Bay, we reach the River Gannel which can be crossed by ferry (789612) to Newquay during the holiday season or by wading at low tide. A low tide footbridge exists inland (799611 or 813608), but it is probably best to ask which is the best way to cross the river at the time. Pick the path up on the other side of Newquay at Watergate Bay, and continue past the amazing rock formations at Bedruthan Steps, around Trevose Head with its lighthouse, and then past Harlyn Bay and Trevone. Stay north-east to Stepper Point and along the west edge of the estuary into Padstow. Take the ferry from here to Rock across the River

Camel. The path then runs along the estuary through Polzeath to the cliffs around Pentire Point.

Just north of Pentire Point at Port Quinn (972805) there is a diversion from the path: follow footpath number 34 from Port Quinn east past the Roascarrock Farm until the junction with path number 16 (at 991805). Follow path number 16 into Pine Haven (989809), just west of Port Isaac. Continue along the coast path Port Isaac through Tintagel (H), and Boscastle (H), after which the going becomes quite challenging. There is easier terrain at Widemouth Sand and Bude, and then once again the path runs over high cliffs and through rugged terrain ending north of Bude at Marsland Mouth.

There are two other route detours as of this writing. One is between Porthpean, (031503), and Pentewan, (021472). From Porthpean take a path south (to 029493) and from there to a road south-east to Trenarren, (033487). From here, take a path (to 025483) and a road from there west into Pentewan.

The other detour is between two points just to the east of Millendreath Beach: (287545 to 276543). To avoid this section, take the coast road from Seaton Beach, (305544), west to Millendreath Beach, (269542).

WALKS ON THE MOORS

The moors of the West Country offer a really special type of walking and hiking country. The moors are largely open, peaty country—Dartmoor even more so than Exmoor. With the aid of a good map, common sense and a compass, you can test your navigation skills on waymarked paths, or make your way on your own paths across the open moor.

There is some danger for inexperienced walkers on the moors, especially because of the cantankerous weather conditions. Fine weather at the beginning of your hike could turn into rain by the end of it. There is little shelter away from the roads, so you should always carry a waterproof with you and check the weather forecast in the paper before you set out. Exposure is no joke—it can happen even in the middle of the summer, and it can kill. If caught out in the weather, watch out for the danger signs of exposure; they are listed on page 217.

I give only two hiking routes, one for each moor. Other routes that you may want to try on Dartmoor are: the Abbots Way between Yelverston and Buckfastleigh; the Mariner's Way from Natsworthy Gate to Throwleigh; and the Lich Way from Bellever to Lydford (the Lich Way was used to carry the dead for burial at Lydford church in medieval times). A good map for Dartmoor is the old One-Inch Ordnance Survey map called the *Dartmoor Tourist Map,* or in the new 1:50,000 Series, there are numbers 202 and 191.

A walk on Exmoor which you may enjoy is an excursion into the "Doone" Valley between Oare and Simonsbath, or via Dunkery Beacon from the coast south to Exford. Use Ordnance Survey maps in the 1:50,000 Series 180 and 181.

   4. *Dartmoor Walk: Postbridge to Dartmeet and back (9 miles)*
From Postbridge head south on a bridleway marked LB 18 (the "L" means Lydford, referring to the general area of the path; "B" means bridleway; "F" means footpath). This takes you to Bellever (H) along the edge of a forest plantation. Bellever is a Forestry Commission village. Go east from here on the main road until just before Bellever Bridge, then south along the East Dart River along a bridleway called the Forest Ride to Laughter Hole Farm, and south-east from there on the LB25 for one mile to Babeny. From here continue south on another bridleway, LB26, along the East Dart River till you come to a minor road a few hundred yards past Brimpts Farm. Turn left on to this road for Dartmeet, close by, a pretty little village in the middle of the moor.

From Dartmeet you go back on to the main road, west, to Huccaby Cottage where you take a bridleway, LB20, north-west over open moorland to the rocks of Huccaby Tor, passing Huccaby Ring on the way; continue north past the large standing stone at Outer Huccaby Ring. After three quarters of a mile, you will pass another stone row just behind Laughter Tor. Continue going north and you will come to Bellever Tor, a little off the bridleway. This is one of the best vantage points in the moor and you may want to climb it to see the views.

At this point, another path joins the bridleway, and you can either continue on the LB20 north-east for Bellever and thence north by the LB18 to Postbridge; or, by by-passing Bellever, you can take the footpath, LF24, from Bellever Tor north through the forest to Postbridge.

5. *Exmoor Walk: Minehead to Lynmouth and Lynton (15 miles)*

This is part of the incomplete Somerset and North Devon Coast Path, which in turn will be part of the Southwest Peninsula Coast Path.

The path begins just south of the harbour at Minehead (H) and climbs to North Hill; from here it passes Selworthy Beacon, from which you may want to make a detour to the left, south on a path through woodland to the little village of Selworthy. This is one of the prettiest villages in the area, with thatched cottages, a fifteenth century tithe barn and a Perpendicular church (by which is meant Perpendicular Gothic, a style of church architecture from the fifteenth century with many vertical lines, as, for example, at Westminster). The path comes into Selworthy just behind the church after crossing the new Scenic Road.

Re-trace your steps out to Selworthy Beacon and continue left, west, on the coast path to Hurtstone Point (there is an alternative route behind this one for those who do not want to go out to the windy point). You descend into Bissington which is another very pretty village. The path rejoins the coast here and follows low-lying land to Porlock Weir.

From Porlock Weir, the path again climbs gradually along the edge of Yearner Wood to continue high up over the sea through Silcombe, Broomstreet and Yenworthy to the Devon boundary at County Gate. The path crosses the A39 road here and skirts the south side of Old Barrow Hill, passing along the fine cliffs through Kipscombe Enclosure, the Foreland and over Butter Hill to Countisbury Church. For those who wish to avoid the Foreland, there is an alternate route over Countisbury Common.

West of Countisbury the path crosses the A39 again to Wind Hill and then descends into the twin resorts of Lynton and Lynmouth (H).

FOUR
The Heart of England

The time of life is short;
To spend that shortness basely
were too long.

WILLIAM SHAKESPEARE: Henry IV, Part 1

To the immediate north-west of London lies the Heart of England, up the Thames Valley to Oxford, and from Oxford north into the Cotswolds and to Stratford-upon-Avon—Shakespeare's country. From there this area stretches west to the Severn Valley and to the Wye Valley. I call this the Heart of England not because it is the industrial pulse-beat of the nation, nor because it is the nation's population centre. It is neither; but, for me, this area *is* England in miniature. If you had only two weeks to spend in England, I would say: spend it here. Of course there will be crowds at Stratford elbowing in line to get tickets for the *Merchant of Venice*; and everyone sends a postcard home from Broadway in the Cotswolds. But at the same time there are quiet country lanes leading into villages of yellow stone on the River Windrush in the Cotswolds; there are the colleges of Oxford which were old already when America was discovered; and there are Tudor and half-timber buildings, so lovely that they must charm even the most jaded of travellers.

This area, more than any other I shall deal with, exemplifies my theory of seeing infinity in a half-mile by really becoming aware of the diversity around you. And, for me, nothing symbolizes this Blakean notion better than the Model Village at Bourton-on-the-Water, itself a miniature Venice on the shallow Windrush River.

At Bourton-on-the-Water, a tiny Cotswold village, there is a model of the village made to one-ninth the scale of the actual village. And within this model is a faithful reproduction of the Model Village; and within this yet another model, and so on, the models becoming smaller and smaller inside one another like Hungarian dolls. And that is precisely the feeling you get as you

roam through this part of England. At first sight this area is just
like the pictures you saw when you first learned geography and it is
all so well manicured that you can hardly believe it is real; and then
your eye adjusts to the amazing variety within such a small area,
just as it does to the model within model. You realize that you
could probably spend several months just walking and riding the
lanes of the Cotswolds, and still not see it all.

You will be going through rolling country and lanes can be used
to great advantage in bike tours, getting you out of the traffic so
that you can enjoy the countryside. There are two bike tours
covering around one hundred miles each, and one long distance
path of eighty-five miles. There are also many shorter walks of
from two to twenty miles. The Cotswolds especially, with the aid
of Ordnance Survey maps, are a walker's paradise with public
footpaths from every little village to the next. It is the perfect area
to try out your own route planning.

The bike routes in the Heart of England are covered by map 13
in the Ordnance Survey Quarter-Inch Series, and by maps 13, 14,
18 and 19 in the Bartholomew 1:100,000 Series.

BIKING

OXFORD, THE COTSWOLDS and
SHAKESPEARE COUNTRY
(130 miles)

This tour takes you from the university town of Oxford north to a
great palace on the edge of the Cotswolds and then through that
beautiful region which was once the wool centre of ancient
Europe. After criss-crossing the Cotswolds, passing through many
lovely villages and seeing plenty of the sheep, stone buildings and
walls that typify the region, the tour heads north for Stratford-
upon-Avon and a tour around Shakespeare's home country.

A word of warning about public transport in the Cotswolds for
those who plan to be on foot—there is not much public transport:
the bus service is irregular at best in the heart of the Cotswolds and
there are no trains. You will either have to try your hand at
hitching or resolve to hike the whole area. Stow-on-the-Wold is
one of the better touring centres as is Cheltenham; both have a

fairly regular bus service, but inter-village bus service is more
difficult, though in a way this can be a blessing, as distances are
not great and you are forced to get out and see the country.

Oxford to Stow-on-the-Wold (40 miles)

Oxford (LCH) is the name of the city and the university. Look
around some of the old colleges—especially Magdalen with its
tower, Christ Church, Merton, All Souls, Balliol, and Trinity.
There is also the Bodleian Library to see and the Ashmolean
Museum which has a large collection of Minoan artifacts from Sir
Arthur Evans' digs at Knossos. Go to Blackwell's in Broad Street
to see what is probably the largest bookshop in the world. Go
punting on the Thames and climb to the top of the tower at
Carfax, once part of St Michael's Church, for views of the city and
surrounding countryside. This should keep any visitor busy for a
couple of days and they will be days well spent.

Head north from Oxford on the A4144 which leads on to the
A34 for Woodstock (L). This was once a hunting lodge on the edge
of King Alfred's Forest; its name means "woody place" in Old
English, but those woods are long gone now. More important for
the tourist today, on the left-hand side of the road coming into the
town, is Blenheim Palace, birthplace of Winston Churchill (his
grave is nearby in Bladon Churchyard just outside the park). The
palace alone covers over three acres, making it the largest palace in
Europe. It has been in the Churchill family since the early
eighteenth century when Queen Anne presented it to John
Churchill, first Duke of Marlborough, to commemorate his
victory over the French at Blenheim. It is said that the great
landscape architect, Capability Brown, laid out the magnificent
gardens to portray the plan of campaign at the battle of Blenheim.

From Woodstock continue north on the A34 for a couple of
miles until you reach the B4437 turning to the left for Charlbury
(H). Continue west on this road till it meets the A361 where you
turn left again, south, into Burford (L). This is an ancient
crossroads town and you can still see evidence of the coaching days
in some of the old inns on Sheep Street.

From Burford take the B4425 west for one mile and then bear
right on a minor road for Little Barrington where you cross the
Windrush River and continue north through Great Barrington.
These two villages are just one example of many twin villages in
the Cotswolds, one prettier than the next it seems, and most with
fine little churches. Continue north and then branch left, north-

west, for Great Rissington, another of the twin villages and stay on this road for Bourton-on-the-Water (L). This is the home of the Model Village mentioned in the introduction to this chapter and it really is fascinating to see; it is also a holiday centre, a busy little place that verges on being over-quaint.

From Bourton cross the A429 going north-west on to a minor road for the Slaughters. There is a right turn off this first minor road going north-east for Upper Slaughter. Have a cream tea at Keynstons Hay Tea Room just above Upper Slaughter on this road. From Upper Slaughter it is possible to make a loop going south-east for Lower Slaughter. The Slaughters are good examples of Cotswold villages which were built around a church and manor.

From Lower Slaughter take a minor road north-east to meet the A436 on which you turn right to head for Stow-on-the-Wold (LH). This is an untypical Cotswold town in some ways: firstly it is built on a hill instead of nestled in a little river valley and secondly it has a market place in the centre; but that does not mean it is not stone-built and lovely. Stow was once a great trade centre for all Europe. Defoe recorded that at one trade fair, 20,000 sheep were sold! There is a good church and some great antique shops. Stow is a good touring centre for the Cotswolds, especially for bikers and hikers: the fine hostel is right in the middle of the town in the old market place; there is a bike rental shop almost next door, plenty of B and Bs, good restaurants and pubs. The hostel warden rents maps of the area and there are many good walks (see under *Hiking*).

Stow-on-the-Wold to Stratford-upon-Avon (35 miles)

From Stow take the A436 and turn right at the Naunton turning, looping across the Windrush and then taking a hard right past Naunton on to a minor road going north through Barton, past the open country around Temple Guiting and across the B4077 into Snowshill just south of Broadway.

At Snowshill you should see the Tudor manor house which houses a fine collection of antique curios, including musical instruments, bicycles and Japanese armour. The collection is open to the public every day except Mondays and Tuesdays in summer and is so vast that the person who collected it all eventually had to move out because there was no room for him.

From here continue north into Broadway (L), *the* tourist centre of the Cotswolds, but still a beautiful little town, perhaps best seen in the early morning. This was a traffic centre in the time of Cromwell, but with the advent of the railway it sank into

The Heart of England

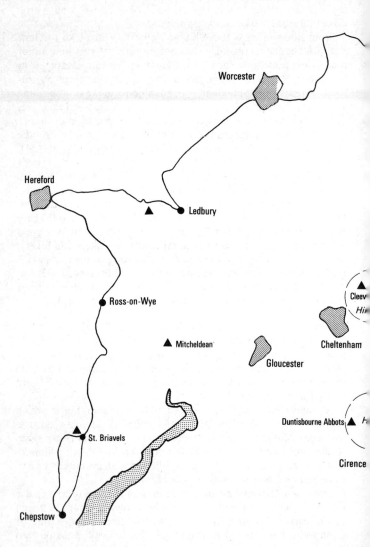

Worcester

Hereford

Ledbury

Ross-on-Wye

Cleev
Hi

Cheltenham

Mitcheldean

Gloucester

Duntisbourne Abbots
H

St. Briavels

Cirence

Chepstow

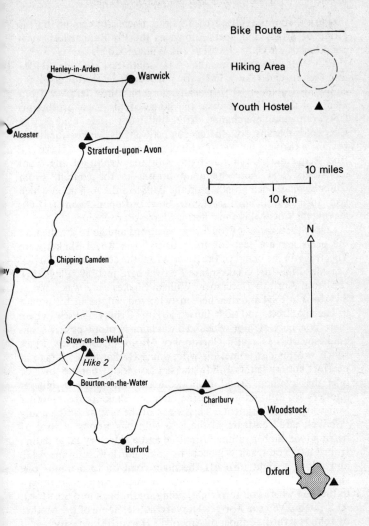

Bike Route ——————

Hiking Area ⟨ ⟩

Youth Hostel ▲

| 0 | | 10 miles |
| 0 | | 10 km |

N

Henley-in-Arden
Warwick
Alcester
▲
Stratford-upon-Avon
Chipping Camden
ay
Stow-on-the-Wold
▲
Hike 2
Bourton-on-the-Water
▲
Charlbury
Woodstock
Burford
Oxford
▲

obscurity. It was re-discovered in the nineteenth century by the group of artists and poets known as the Pre-Raphaelites, such people as Dante Gabriel Rosetti and William Morris.

From Broadway take the A44 south-east to the B4081 intersection and take a left turn north-east on to this road for Chipping Campden (L), a really gorgeous little leftover from medieval times. It was once the home of the most prosperous Cotswold wool merchants. After the wool trade died in the Cotswolds because of stiffer competition elsewhere, the town became a thriving market—"chipping" means market. There is a fine Perpendicular church built with the wealth of the wool merchants, and there are good brasses in the church. From Chipping Campden go north on the B4081 to the A46 upon which you turn right, north-east, to Stratford-upon-Avon (HLC), leaving the Cotswolds and entering Shakespeare country.

Ignore the swarms of tourists at Stratford and go to the theatre, the plays are not just for the tourists. The Royal Shakespeare Theatre is on the banks of the River Avon; the actor David Garrick organized the first Shakespeare Festival here in 1769. Plays now run from April to December. William Shakespeare was born at Stratford in 1564 and died here in 1616; you can see his birthplace in Henley Street, and he is buried at Holy Trinity Church (where there is a bust of him which critics claim is proof positive that Shakespeare was really Christopher Marlowe). See New Place which was his last home; his wife, Anne Hathaway's, cottage at nearby Shottery (either follow the signs on foot from the town or take the Evesham Road from Rother Street, turning right at Shottery Road); and also see the home of Shakespeare's mother Mary Arden, at Wilmcote. This is one of the best of all the many "Shakespeare" cottages in the area with oak beams, a roof of herringbone timber, a huge fireplace and a refectory table dating from 1480. You reach Wilmcote by going north-west on the A422 and taking a right turn off the main road on to a minor one signposted to Billesley. Loop through Wilmcote then go north-east to the A34 where you turn right, going south, back into Stratford. At Stratford you can also see Harvard house, home of the Mother of John Harvard, founder of America's Harvard University.

Stratford-upon-Avon to Alcester (30 miles)

From Stratford take a minor road through Alveston where the Stratford hostel is located; this joins up with the A429 where you turn left, going north into Warwick (LC). Warwick has one of the finest castles in England standing on a rocky site overlooking the River Avon. There are rows of black and white Tudor houses to be seen in Mill Street as well as the Beauchamp Chapel and the Doll Museum in Castle Street.

From Warwick take the minor road west through Clavendon for Henley-in-Arden (LC). A one-time stronghold of Plantagenet power, this is a fine old market town with a good Guild Hall. Try the White Swan, the Old George or the Blue Bell Inn for a pint. From Henley take the A34 south for two miles and then bear right, south-west on the B4089 for Alcester, a nice old town with many timber-framed buildings. Once you begin heading west out of Alcester, you officially leave Shakespeare country and have come nearly to the end of the first bike tour of this region. The next tour starts at Worcester and travels near the Malvern Hills west to Hereford and south into the Wye Valley. The following twenty-five mile tour links up the two tours.

Alcester to Worcester (25 miles)

From Alcester take the B4090 north-west through Feckenham then take a hard left south on a minor road through Crowley to the A422 upon which you turn right, west, into Worcester (CL).

Worcester is a city much spoiled by modern development but there is still some of its former Tudor charm left. It is one of the three cathedral cities of the west, the other two are Gloucester and Hereford. The cathedral at Worcester is excellent: begun in 1084, it was added to during every succeeding architectural period. Thus you can trace the development of style from Norman through Early English Gothic to Perpendicular Gothic all in this one building.

HEREFORDSHIRE and THE WYE VALLEY
(90 miles)

Worcester to Hereford (35 miles)

From Worcester take the A4103 south-west out of town towards Hereford, but take a minor road left, south, for Bosbury after about ten miles. From Bosbury continue south-east into Ledbury (HL), the birthplace of the poet John Masefield and a neat little town with top-heavy black and white buildings leaning on oak pillars. This is a good centre for walking in the Malvern Hills to the north. From Ledbury take the A438 west to Hereford (L), the

second cathedral city in the West. Hereford is an ancient town
dating back to the seventh century. Situated on the River Wye, the
town is noted for the salmon caught locally in that river. (See
Chapter Seven for an alternative route north to Chester which by-
passes Wales.)

Hereford to Goodrich (25 miles)

From Hereford take a minor road south-east through Mordiford
on the east side of the River Wye and follow the Wye through
Fownhope where you take another minor road to the right, south,
staying close to the river, through Howcaple, Brempton Abbots
and across the A40 into Ross-on-Wye (CL). This is an old market
town built on a wooded cliff; it is a centre for travels into the Wye
Valley and the Forest of Dean. Take a minor road south out of
Ross toward Goodrich. This road joins the B4228 after a few miles
and continues south near Goodrich—you can go into Goodrich
though this tour is not routed through the town, but on the B4228
which takes you past the hostel at Welsh Bicknor.

Goodrich to Chepstow (25 miles)

Continue south on the B4228 into the Forest of Dean, an old royal
hunting forest preserved now for the public instead of for royalty.
It is situated on a high plateau between the Severn and Wye Rivers
with many enchanting little roads and hiking paths (see under
Hiking) criss-crossing it. Make some detours into the heart of the
Forest or just continue to St Briavels (H) on the B4228 going
south. Staying on this road you will go through Hewelsfield and
into Chepstow (LCH).

However, there is an alternate route for part of this journey
from St Briavels going south-west on a minor road to cross the
Wye and Offa's Dyke (see under *Hiking*). Continue into East
Wales to the A466 upon which you turn left, south, to go through
the lovely picture postcard village of Tintern. Nearby is Tintern
Abbey, the same ruin about which Wordsworth wrote his famous
Lines. This was a great Cistercian Abbey in 1131, and is now a
magnificent skeleton amid the trees, with green grass growing in
the nave.

Continue south into Chepstow and the end of the route.
Chepstow is set near the conflux of the Wye and the Severn and is
a pretty, yet illusive sort of town with a great bulldog of a Norman
castle in ruins.

HIKING

NOTE: Offa's Dyke Path, a difficult 168-mile long-distance route running north to south along the entire length of the Welsh border, actually intersects the end of the last bike route. It may be a good opportunity therefore for some hiking. However, as most of this path is in the Welsh touring area, it is described in Chapter Five.

THE RIDGEWAY PATH
(85 miles)

This route makes use of the ancient trackways which formed part of the pre-historic route from the Devon coast to East Anglia. The path stays on the crest of the Berkshire and Marlborough Downs and the Chiltern Hills. Like the analogous routes on the ridges of the North and South Downs, this trackway offered ancient traders a dry and easily navigated passage on their journeys between the Continent and Ireland.

A good book about the Ridgeway, in an archaeological vein, is *The Oldest Road—An Exploration of the Ridgeway,* by Fay Godwin and J. R. L. Anderson. Ordnance Survey maps in the 1:50,000 Series are 173, 174, 175 and 165. The way is marked with acorn and oak signposts or low stone plinths. The Ridgeway is, after the South Downs Way, the easiest of the long distance paths; perfect for the novice and the experienced walker alike. The first part of the path from Overton Hill to Streatley is bridleway, suitable for cyclists and horse-riders as well as walkers. This area contains many Bronze and Iron Age monuments and remains—religious monuments, burial places, fortifications and habitations from two to three thousand years old. East of Streatley the Ridgeway is mostly footpath, quiet walking country, with good views. The route passes through many villages, and there are also a few hostels on the route so that accommodation is no great problem. However, if you are planning to do the whole route, I would advise carrying camping gear.

1. *Overton Hill to Ivinghoe Beacon (85 miles)*
This route starts at the west end of the Ridgeway leaving the A4 at Overton Hill about four miles west of Marlborough (L) and two miles east of Avebury. The path follows the ridge north across

Overton Down and is then met by a track that comes up from the
Stone Circle at Avebury. If you are starting at Avebury you follow
a disused road from near the bus stop—ask anyone in Avebury for
directions to the Ridgeway.

At Hackpen Hill the path reaches the nine hundred foot level
and then continues east along the southern boundary of Barbury
Castle Park where there are some good views. The ancient
Ridgeway here crosses lower ground and is a paved road until
Liddington Castle, so a detour from the ancient path is given,
taking you south-east along Smeathe's Ridge to cross the River
Og, just south of Ogbourne St George; then turning back north
along the escarpment to rejoin the Ridgeway where it crosses the
A419. The route is still a paved road for a while across the
Wanborough Plain as far as Fox Hill where it crosses the M4
motorway. The path continues from Fox Hill climbing on to the
Downs, crossing the boundary of Oxfordshire and Wiltshire near
Bishopstone.

The next twenty-three miles take you through Oxfordshire and
Berkshire past many archaeological sites: Alfred's Castle,
Wayland Smith's Cave, a Bronze Age dolmen group, past
Bardwell Camp, Uffington Castle, and White Horse Hill. Then the
path continues south-east past Segsbury Camp and Lowbury Hill,
crossing downland up to seven hundred feet high and giving good
views—especially over the Vale of the White Horse. Villages
within easy reach are: Compton Beauchamp, Letcombe Bassett,
Letcombe Regis, Chilton, East Ilsley, Blewbury, and Aston
Tirrold. At Streatley (H) the path crosses the River Thames to
Goring via a bridge road and returns into Oxfordshire.

The path from Goring goes north for about six miles following
the bank of the Thames to Mongewell Park where it turns east to
follow an ancient earthwork, known as Grim's Ditch, to the village
of Nuffield. The path goes over Nuffield Common, through
Ewelme Park and across Swyncombe Downs then drops down to
join the Icknield Way near the village of Britwell.

The Icknield Way is the oldest trackway in Europe (see the
discussion of the ley systems on page 46). The Icknield Way
extends from Norfolk to the Wiltshire border; much of it was
incorporated into the Roman road system, and many miles of this
ancient pathway are, today, paved road. You follow the Icknield
Way for about ten miles and it is a broad path offering good views.
Go north-east either through or near Ewelme, Watlington,
Lewknor, Aston Rowant, and Chinnor as far as the county

boundary with Buckinghamshire at Hampton Wainhill.

There is another detour which starts in Buckinghamshire where more of the old track is paved road. The path turns south-east from Hampton Wainhill and climbs over Lodge Hill, away from the Icknield Way. It then drops down to cross a railway line and road just south of Princes Risborough, where the path rejoins the Icknield Way for a short distance before it climbs over Whiteleaf Hill to Lower Cadsden. The path continues in a north-east direction past Chequers Estate, Lodge Hill, Coombe Hill (825 feet), and Bacombe Hill; then the path drops down into Wendover (H nearby at Lee Gate). From here the path goes north-east towards Tring cutting through heavily wooded country at Cocks Hill and across a strip of Hertfordshire near Pendley Manor, then crossing a railway line near Tring Station. The path ascends the wooded slopes of Aldbury Nowers and re-enters Buckinghamshire at Pitstone Hill. The last section of the path goes north over lovely downland to Ivinghoe Beacon with a hostel at nearby Ivinghoe.

This route can obviously be walked the other way, starting from the east end (not far from London).

WALKS IN THE COTSWOLDS

There are some excellent books and pamphlets about hiking in the Cotswolds, all giving minute instructions about which path to take over which turn-stile, etc. But personally, I find these very detailed instructions difficult to use because they are so complicated. However, if you do not know the way or are not using a map then these minute descriptions are almost essential if you are going to stay on public rights of way. I give here only a few simple hiking routes that stay mainly on roads and bridleways for ease of direction. The roads are minor roads with little traffic, yet paved nonetheless. It will be up to you to discover, with the help of maps, more walks and paths for your own enjoyment. For example, there is an excellent four to five day walk right across the Cotswolds following footpaths all the way, and going to each of the three hostels in the area. There is not just one way to do this hike, but many. All you have to do is get the Ordnance Survey map 163 in the 1:50,000 Series and follow the red, dotted lines. By following those lines and asking people in the villages you pass through for paths leading to the next village, you will not need detailed directions from a book.

There is a long distance path in the Cotswolds that stretches from Bath to Chipping Campden. Maps covering the route in the 1:50,000 Ordnance Survey Series are 173, 163 and 150. Good stretches for short walks along this path are near Wootton-under-Edge, Stroud, Painswick, Cleeve Hill (part of which is included below), and Broadway.

Also see under *Biking* in this chapter for a discussion of public transport problems encountered in the Cotswolds.

The following are four separate one-day walks to be done from the hostels in the Cotswolds.

1 & 2. *Walks around Stow-on-the-Wold (8 miles each)*

The first route goes over some country already seen on the bike tour, (see page 77). Take the bus from Stow to Bourton-on-the-Water, and from Bourton follow the routes given in the biking section. The route takes you through the lovely twin villages of the Slaughters and back to Stow by minor roads, or you can go out to the A429 and catch a bus back to Stow. But be sure to check the bus times from and to Stow-on-the-Wold before leaving. You can rent a map from the warden at the Stow Hostel.

Another route of about seven to eight miles takes you north-east out of Stow on a tiny road from the back of the hostel to Broadwell Hill and from there due north on the same unpaved road to Broadwell. From Broadwell you head south-east on a minor road past Sydenham Farm to Oddington, where there is a pottery works and a good chance to see some local craftsmanship. From Oddington you take a footpath from the south-west end of the village across fields to the B4450 and take a left turn on that road, south, for a few hundred yards to another minor road going to Icomb. From Icomb there is a narrow little road going north over Maugersbury Hill, through Oxlease, across some railway lines and into Maugersbury. From there it is a quarter of a mile north-west on another minor road for Stow. This route takes you through pleasant countryside and gives you a chance to get off the roads.

3. *A Walk from Duntisbourne Abbots Hostel to Chedworth Roman Villa (7 miles)*

There are many Roman villa sites in the Cotswold county of Gloucestershire. From the first century to the fourth century AD the Roman influence in this area manifested itself in a bizarre, anachronistic suburbia, fifteen hundred years before its time.

Great country houses arose, self-sufficient, raising their own crops, and having central heating, beautiful mosaics, and lavish baths. After the collapse of the Roman Empire and the ensuing raids of the Saxons, Angles and a host of others into England, there was a period of chaos, since called the Dark Ages. This was the age of Arthur and also the time when these great Roman villas fell into ruin. Roving bands of marauders moved into the deserted villas for a night, or a month, lighting cooking-fires on the mosaics and destroying anything they could find.

Chedworth is a classic example of a Romano-British villa. Almost the whole of the main building complex is visible, with two suites of baths, and evidence of the Roman form of heating with hypocausts laid between the short tile columns that supported the floor. There are several good mosaics, one with figures of nymphs and satyrs and figures of the four seasons in the corners; there is also a nymphaeum, an ornamental fountain structure built over a spring. Finds from the excavations are displayed in the site museum which is open every day except Monday.

To get to Chedworth from the hostel (the hostel is five miles north-west of Cirencester), you take the minor road east out of the village to the A417 and turn right, south-east for a few hundred yards—this is the Ermin Way, an old straight-as-an-arrow Roman road. Stay on this till you come to a minor road on the left leading to Woodmancote. Proceed through Woodmancote and on to another minor road north-east going through Old Park and crossing the A435 to Rendcomb. From Rendcomb there is an unpaved road leading north-east across a paved road and past a long barrow on the right about one and a half miles from Rendcomb. Turn left on to another minor road for Chedworth; proceed through the village and follow the footpath signs to the villa which is about one mile away to the north, through Chedworth Woods.

From Chedworth you can either return to the hostel or keep going perhaps into Northleach for the night, and continue on to Stow or Cheltenham the next day.

4. *A Walk Around Cleeve Hill (7 miles)*

Cleeve Hill Hostel is situated three to four miles north-east of Cheltenham. Cheltenham is a one time Georgian spa with West-End style shops and a Victorian atmosphere. The route that follows takes you from the hostel to the long barrow tomb at Belas Knap and back.

Take the footpath to the immediate north of the hostel and follow it in a north-east direction for five hundred yards where it meets an unpaved little road going north-south. Turn right going south past the golf course and over Cleeve Common and take the left fork where the path divides a few hundred yards over the Common. Keep going in a south-east direction and then an east direction to Wontley Farm where you take a hard left going north-east till you meet a footpath going off to the right to Belas Knap about five hundred yards away. As this long barrow is on a hillside and looks rather like a wasps' nest on the ground, it would be hard to miss it. The tomb was built at about the same time as the pyramids of Egypt and when the communal burial chamber was opened in 1863, about thirty skeletons were found. The barrow has been restored and you can explore the interior. Be sure to take a close look at the stone work and see how much it resembles modern-day stone work in the Cotswolds.

From Belas Knap go back out to the unpaved road via the footpath and turn right, going north, for a quarter of a mile, take the left turn to the west to skirt Corndean Hall. Continue west for another half mile till the unpaved road becomes a public bridleway which you follow north-west to Postlip Hall and via footpaths skirting the golf course to meet the same little road upon which you started. Turn left going first west and then south for the remaining one mile to the hostel.

WALKS IN THE FOREST OF DEAN

The Forest of Dean is on a high plateau between the Severn and Wye rivers and was once a royal hunting preserve. It is now a nature reserve for the public. There are many good hiking trails and small roads criss-crossing the Forest and as many as nine well-marked, short nature trails (two to three miles). There is good bird-watching in the Forest with the usual array of woodland birds, plus buzzards, ravens and nightjars.

The Speech House Forest Trail, a three-mile walk, begins either at Speech House or at Beechenhurst Picnic Place. Another good nature trail, also a three-mile walk, is the Edge End Trail, beginning at the Edge End Picnic Place. The trails are simple to follow and well marked. For other hikes in the Forest consult Ordnance Survey map 162 in the 1:50,000 Series.

FIVE

Wales

One road leads to London,
One road runs to Wales
Any road leads me seawards
To the white dipping sails.

JOHN MASEFIELD: Roadways

Wales is one of the best, most varied touring areas in Britain but for many bikers and hikers its hills and mountains may be too much. It is not for the beginner; in some regions, such as Snowdonia, there is no way to avoid a long uphill pull but remember: once you're up, you're up.

The two bike routes given here are designed for the biker who wants to cross at Fishguard for Ireland, landing at Rosslare, and then cross back from Dublin to Holyhead. Thus, there is a south bike route into, and a north bike route out of Wales. If you are not planning to go to Ireland and if you want to avoid the hilly country of Wales there is a route along the border counties from Hereford to Chester included in the next chapter.

Wales can be wet in summer so be sure to carry rain gear. There is good fishing on the Usk, Wye, Severn, Towy and Dwyfd Rivers; you can catch perch in Lake Trawsfynydd, pike in Lake Langorse and in the Brecon Beacons and bream in the Lower Dee River.

Wales is a land of castles and poetry. It is also a mecca for the hill walker and climber. There are caves, coal and Dylan Thomas—not to mention towns with names that measure in feet. The Welsh language is still alive and well, for Wales is definitely not England and the ancient Celtic traditions hold out here as they do in Ireland, Cornwall and parts of Scotland.

Overleaf is a short glossary of Welsh words you may need, for although most Welsh people speak English, many signs and place-names are in Welsh:

aber: mouth of a river or stream
afon: river
bach: small
ban: high place or peak
bedd: grave
brynn: hill
bwlch: pass, gap
caer: fort
carreg, carrig (pl): stone
capel: chapel
castel: castle
cefn: cefnydd (pl): ridge
coed: wood, trees
craig: rock
cwm: valley, dale
dinas: city, fort
dyffryn: valley
eglwys: church

eisteddfod: contest of music and poetry
garth: enclosure
glyn: deep valley, glen
hafod: summer residence
hendre: winter residence
heol: road
llwybr: path
llyn: lake
mawr: great, big
newydd: new
pen, pennau (pl): end, top, head, edge
plas: mansion
tan, dan: under, beneath
traeth: beach
trum: trumiau (pl): ridge
ty: house
ynys: island

I describe two bike routes in Wales, one in the north and one in the south, but this does not mean that mid-Wales, which has the coast, the lakes, forest walks and nature trails, is not also worth a visit. There is pony trekking and there are places to fish all over Wales. Also in mid-Wales, you can hire a pony caravan and wander through the mountain scenery of the Ystwyth and Rheidol Rivers.

For hikers I describe two fairly difficult long-distance paths. There is one in the west along Offa's Dyke which goes all the way from the Dee to the Severn estuary from north to south along the border with England. The other is on the south-west coast in the Pembrokeshire National Park. There is also good hill walking in the Snowdonia National Park in the north and in the Brecon Beacons National Park in the south.

The bike routes in Wales are covered by maps 10 and 12 in the Ordnance Survey Quarter-Inch Series, and by maps 11, 12, 13, 17 (South), 23, 27 and 28 (North) in the Bartholomew 1:100,000 Series.

BIKING

The South: CHEPSTOW to FISHGUARD
(130 miles)

Chepstow to Brecon (35 miles)

This southern route is not as hilly or mountainous as the northern one. The first part takes you to Brecon, a centre for hiking in the Brecon Beacons (see under *Hiking*).

From Chepstow (LCH), a picturesque town with a Norman castle, go west on the B4235 for Usk. From Usk continue north on the A471 which joins up with the A40 going north-west through Abergavenny (L) with its twelfth century castle. Continue west on the A4077 (across the river and parallel with the A40, the main road through South Wales). The A4077 becomes the B4558 just across the River Usk from Crickhowell (HL) and continues west into Brecon (HL). This is a busy market town with a castle and a cathedral, the gateway to the Brecon Beacons mountains and park.

Brecon to Carmarthen (40 miles)

From Brecon continue west on the A40 for about ten miles to Trecastle where you turn left on to a minor road, south-west towards Trapp via the hostel at Llandeusant and across the A4069. From Trapp continue on a minor road south-west through Llandebie and from there take another minor road through Penygroes till you meet the junction with the A476 where you turn left to go south for a mile into Cross Hands. From there take the A48 north-west into Carmarthen (L), which has a skeleton of a castle on the cliff, the remains of what was once the home of the princes of South Wales. There is also a legend that Merlin was born at Carmarthen; the Old Oak in Priory Street is associated with the magician and legend tells how Merlin prophesied that when the oak fell the town would fall also. Both, however, still stand.

Carmarthen to Haverfordwest (35 miles)

Take the A40 west out of Carmarthen for about ten miles till you reach St Clears where you turn left, south, on to the A4066 to Laugharne (CL), pronounced "Larn". This is one of the finest small towns in Wales, with a twelfth century castle; however, the real attraction of the town is that it was the home of Dylan Thomas. He lived and worked in the Boat House, which is situated

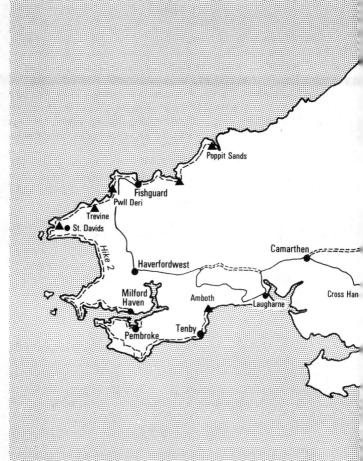

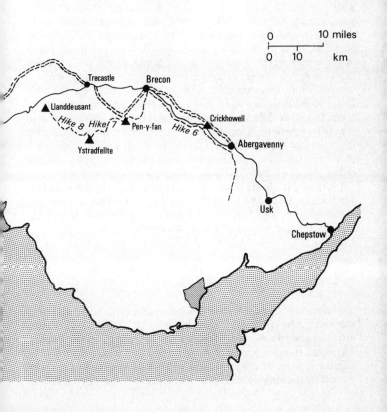

South Wales

Bike Route

Hike Route

Connecting Route

▲ Youth Hostel

N

0 ___ 10 miles
0 ___ 10 ___ km

Trecastle   Brecon
Llanddeusant
Hike 8 Hike 7   Pen-y-fan   Crickhowell
Ystradfellte   Hike 6   Abergavenny

Usk

Chepstow

between the hillside and the river bank, along the cliff walk which starts at the back of the castle. The Boat House is now a Dylan Thomas Museum and well worth a visit; it was here that the poet wrote *Under Milk Wood*; his simple grave is in the local cemetery. You can down a pint to his memory at his favourite drinking spot, Brown's Hotel.

From Laugharne you take a minor road west until it meets the B4314 where you turn right, north-west, through Tavernspite and Narbeth (C) until you meet the A40 once again. Turn left, west, into Haverfordwest (CL), the county town of Pembrokeshire and a good touring centre for the Pembrokeshire National Park (see under *Hiking*).

Haverfordwest to Fishguard (20 miles)

Take the B4330 north out of Haverfordwest for about six miles until you are just beyond Haycastle Cross, then turn right, north, on to a minor road for Castle Morris, cross the A487 for St Nicholas, a sleepy little town which has the finest old petrol pump in the whole world. I am not sure if petrol comes out of it any more—but you can get groceries from the little shop in the petrol station. From here continue north past the turning for the Pwll Deri youth hostel (see under *Hiking*), a good hostel if you want to spend the night isolated on the brink of the world—so near is it to the cliffs. Continue along this minor road, or the lower one nearer the coast past the lighthouse at Strumble Head, and into Goodwick and from there into Fishguard following the main road for this last mile.

Fishguard (L) is the ferry terminus for Ireland, the ferry lands at Rosslare in the south-east of the Republic of Ireland, a three-and-a-quarter hour trip. There is a fine harbour in the lower town here, scene of the film version of *Under Milk Wood*.

The North: HOLYHEAD to CHESTER
(105 miles)

This north route includes two alternate routes which can add to or subtract only ten miles from the overall mileage. The main attraction in the north, as far as I am concerned, is Snowdonia. The route is mountainous, but in the end well worth the toil. The scenery is some of the finest you will see in Britain, so do not be put off by the long uphill climb—there are very few steep gradients but several long, slow uphill stretches; you can always walk your bike when the going gets really tough.

Holyhead to Bangor (25 miles)

Starting on the island of Anglesey from Holyhead (L), which is a major port for Ireland, an industrial town and a holiday resort, you could take the A5 all the way to Bangor; but this road can get hectic with traffic to and from the ferry, so I advise you to take the A5 for a few miles south east to Valley, where you turn left, north-east on to the A5025 to Llanynghenedle, where you turn right, east, on to the B5109 for about fifteen miles to Llangefni. From there take minor roads to Cein and through Penmynydd and then back on to the A5 at the town with fifty-seven letters to its name which means "St Mary's by the White Aspen over the Whirlpool and St Tysilio's by the Red Cave". On maps it is, thankfully, shortened to Llanfair. Look at the nameplate at the station: I have heard that the original nameplate had to be put in a local museum because so many tourists tried to steal it! From here continue south-east across the Menai Suspension Bridge over the Menai Strait, leaving the Island of Anglesey and continuing into Bangor (HCL). The building of the Menai Bridge was begun in 1820; it is half a mile long with a central span of 579 feet. Bangor is a university town and Upper Bangor is definitely the nicest part: there are some fine old houses and pubs and several good Chinese and Indian restaurants. Bangor, under-rated by most travellers, is definitely worth a visit.

Bangor to Capel Curig (30 or 22 miles)

The alternate routes from Bangor are via Caernarvon (thirty miles) or via Llanberis (twenty-two miles).

From Bangor to Caernarvon (CL) take the A487, south, all the way. Caernarvon is near the coast, it has a magnificent castle, supposedly the mightiest in all Europe in the thirteenth century. It was the setting, in 1969, of the investiture of Prince Charles as Prince of Wales. The town is a bustling tourist centre. From Caernarvon you take the A4085 south-east for some six miles into the heart of the Snowdonia National Park to the Snowdon Ranger Hostel, which is a good centre for hill walking set just at the base of Mount Snowdon (see under *Hiking*). From Snowdon continue on the A4085 south-east to Beddgelert which is a splendid mountain town with lots of stone-built inns. You turn left here on to the A498 going north-east past Pen-y-Pass (H) to the junction of

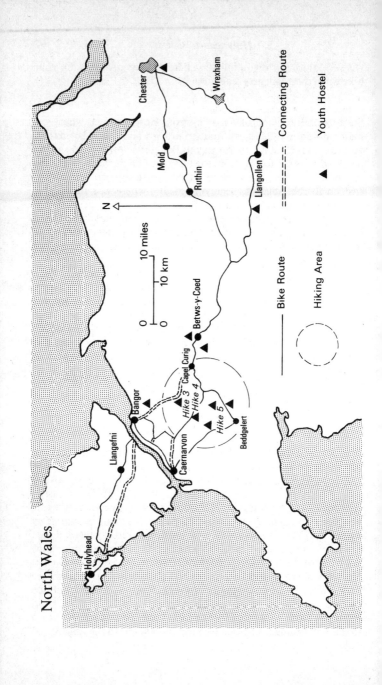

North Wales

N

10 miles
10 km
0

===== Connecting Route
——— Bike Route
▲ Youth Hostel
⌇ Hiking Area

Chester
Wrexham
Mold
Ruthin
Llangollen
Betws-y-Coed
Bangor
Capel Curig
Llangefni
Caernarvon
Holyhead
Beddgelert

Hike 3
Hike 4
Hike 5

the A4086 which you follow east into Capel Curig (H).

For those who want to go straight into Snowdonia and avoid the trip south to Caernarvon, take the A5 from Bangor for a mile and then turn right, south, on the B4409 through Pentir and then turn left, south-east, on to the B4547 for three miles until this road meets the A4086 where you turn left, south-east, to follow that road into Llanberis (LH). This is the official centre for touring in Snowdonia; there is even a narrow-gauge railway to the summit of Mount Snowdon and this is by far the easiest way to ascend the mountain! (see under *Hiking*.) From Llanberis follow the A4086 south-east over Llanberis Pass (1169 feet) and into Capel Curig. This is the home of the National Mountaineering Centre, and there is plenty of rock climbing and also beautiful scenery. Once here, the long, hard pull is over. In fact the hardest part is only a matter of five to six miles and that is before Capel Curig.

Capel Curig to Chester (55 miles)

From Capel Curig you sail downhill on the A5 into Betws-y-Coed (LCH) a lush beauty spot usually packed with tourists; there are some of the best hotels here that I have seen in Wales. The hostel is several miles out of town to the north, at Oaklands. From Betws-y-Coed or from the hostel, take a minor road for Capel Garmon to avoid the traffic on the main road. You join the A5 several miles to the south-east and continue into Cerrigydrudion (C), where the route splits into a north and a south choice.

The choice of the south route would be especially good in early July when there is an International *Eisteddfod* at Llangollen (LH). This town can be reached by continuing on the A5 for about twenty-five miles from Cerrigydrudion. From Llangollen you take the A483 for Wrexham (L), the centre of the North Wales coalfields, an ancient town with the lovely church of St Giles. From Wrexham you can take the A483 north-east into Chester.

However, if you decide on the shorter north route, from Cerrigydrudion you branch left, north-east, on to the B5105 across the Clocaenog Forest to Ruthin (L), which is yet another small town with a castle; also look at the sixteenth century half-timbered Exmewe Hall. From Ruthin continue north-east on the A494 past the hostel at Maeshafn and into Mold. From Mold take a minor road east through Buckley and on to the A55, across the Welsh border and into the walled city of Chester (HCL).

Chester really is a lovely old city; originally a Roman city, it still has the old wall around it, parts of which date from Roman times and other sections from the Middle Ages. There are some two-storey, black and white half-timbered buildings that are now shops; the second floors are connected with one another by means of a long outdoor gallery. See the impressive eleventh century cathedral, the choir is the highpoint, with carved stalls which date from the fourteenth century.

The northern route is about ten miles shorter than the southern route.

HIKING

OFFA'S DYKE LONG DISTANCE PATH
(168 miles)

This is a difficult path running north to south, from Prestatyn on Liverpool Bay in the north to the Sedbury Cliffs near Chepstow on the Severn Estuary in the south. The path runs for sixty miles along the line of a ditch and bank protective dyke built in the eighth century by Offa, King of Mercia, to control his border with the Welsh. The path also connects the medieval market towns which grew up around the castles which were erected by the English as a protective system against marauders from the Welsh Hills.

Little remains of the dyke in Herefordshire, so that another route has been devised over the border hills and the east ridge of the Black Mountains. The Clun Forest in the middle of the route is a lonely upland; the valleys of the Dee and Wye offer some of the easiest stretches through picturesque wooded countryside. The whole route could take from two to three weeks, even when the weather is good. Offa's Dyke path is one of those that is better done in bits and pieces—some stretches coincide quite well with bike routes already given (see the bike route of the Wye Valley in Chapter Four and also the north bike route in this chapter). This is a tough path and you should be reasonably fit before attempting all of it, or even the more difficult stretches. Remember especially the uncertainty of the weather in Wales; and if you are not familiar with the use of compass or do not have one, it would be best not to tackle the Black Mountains or Denbigh Moor.

Ordnance Survey maps in the 1:50,000 Series are 162, 149, 137,

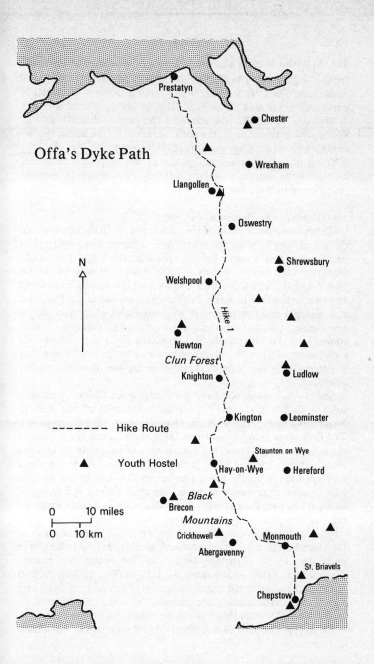

Offa's Dyke Path

N

Prestatyn

● Chester

● Wrexham

Llangollen

● Oswestry

▲ Shrewsbury

Welshpool

Hike 1

▲
●
Newton

Clun Forest

▲
● Ludlow
Knighton

● Kington ● Leominster

▲

Staunton on Wye
Hay-on-Wye ● Hereford

Black
▲
Brecon
Mountains
Crickhowell ▲ ▲ Monmouth ▲
Abergavenny

St. Briavels

Chepstow

– – – – Hike Route

▲ Youth Hostel

0   10 miles
0   10 km

126, 117, which cover the whole length of the path. Good books about the path are, *The Shell Book of Offa's Dyke Path* by Frank Noble, and *The Offa's Dyke Path* by Arthur Roberts. Both can be purchased in the area of the path. The path is signposted with oak or concrete posts with the name of the path in English and/or Welsh. Away from roads, the path is marked by the acorn symbol at places where the hiker might take the wrong path.

There are several hostels along the way and the path is connected by numerous minor roads to villages nearby which provide lodging and public transport.

1. *Prestatyn to Chepstow (168 miles)*

I will begin my description of the path in the north though it would be just as easy to walk the other way, from south to north. The path begins at Prestatyn on the Flintshire coast and goes south along the escarpment of the Clwydian Range, passing by several Iron Age hill forts; there are views west all the way to Snowdonia and east to the Dee Estuary. The path crosses the tiny Alyn River at Llandegla and proceeds over wild moorland which you should avoid unless you are experienced with maps and compass. It then comes into the hills north of Llangollen (HL) and follows the escarpment of Eglwyseg giving more views to the west. From here it descends to the Vale of Llangollen by the Pont-y-Cyssyllte aqueduct.

South from Llangollen the path goes near Chirk Castle and follows Offa's Dyke over the eastern foothills of the Berwyn Mountains giving views of the Oswestry and Shropshire plains. The Dyke here is huge and formidable and you can get an idea of the engineering problem that it must have presented to its builders in the eighth century. The path continues to follow the Dyke through Llanymynech, along the Severn floodbanks and the old Montgomeryshire canal; it crosses the river Severn at Buttington Bridge. The path then ascends Long Mountain to Beacon Ring and then down again to the Montgomery lowland, where the best parts of the earthwork begin. The path traverses the sheep pastures of the Clun Forest, after which you walk along the Dyke to Knighton and almost into Kington before turning south-west toward Gladestry and then south again for Hay-on-Wye, a busy market with some fantastic old coaching inns—try particularly the Three Cocks. Also visit Booth's bookshop—Hay is the only town in the world where the bookshops are bigger than the supermarkets.

From Hay the path climbs steeply up into the Black Mountains, another stretch where compass and map-reading skills are needed. The path stays close to the east edge of these mountains by the hostel at Capel-y-ffin and then takes a south-east turning over mountain moorland to Pandy. From there it passes White Castle in the rolling countryside of Monmouthshire and enters the Wye Valley. The Dyke and the path follow the valley south through woods, with a glimpse of Tintern Abbey below. Alternate routes are from Bigsweir to Brockweir either along the banks of the Wye or along the bank of the Dyke (where river and Dyke diverge). The path ends at Sedbury Cliffs on the Severn near Chepstow (CHL).

PEMBROKESHIRE COAST PATH
(170 miles)

This is a tough path, though not quite so arduous as the Offa's Dyke path. Some of the best scenery in Europe is to be seen on this route—there are some really terrific coastal cliff walks. The coast of the Pembrokeshire National Park is one of the richest areas in Britain for sea-birds; it is also the archaeologist's and geologist's dream.

Use Ordnance Survey maps in the 1:50,000 Series 147, 157, 158. The Countryside Commission has published a book about the path called *The Pembrokeshire Coast Path.* There are numerous hostels and small towns along the route which provide accommodation, but if travelling in the high season, either try to reserve ahead of time if you are relying solely on indoor lodgings, or carry camping equipment with you, because this is a popular area.

The way is marked by signposts, with the words *Coast Path,* where the path leaves or joins roads. Away from the roads, where there is a chance that you may take the wrong turning, the acorn symbol is used to mark the correct path.

2. *Amroth to St Dogmaels (170 miles)*
The coast path can be walked from either north to south or south to north. I describe the route from south to north. The path starts in the south at Amroth where there is an ancient submerged forest revealed only at low tide. From here the path runs along the bay to Saundersfoot (H), a busy harbour with sandy beaches on both sides of the bay. The path continues on to Tenby (L) which is a fairly unspoilt medieval town with narrow streets and a ruined

fourteenth century castle on the hill above the town. The path continues west to the estuary of Milford Haven, a good natural harbour—so good in fact that it has become the home of enormous ugly oil refineries. Before you reach the estuary you must make some detours to avoid Ministry of Defence areas at Penally, Manorbier and Castle Martin. Red warning flags will be flying when firing is taking place but always check locally to make sure. These inland detours are all well signposted.

After you have negotiated the firing ranges you will round the Angle Peninsula and head east by Angle Bay and Pwllcochran to Pembroke Castle, a sturdy Norman building from the eleventh century. From here the path continues across Monkton Bridge to Pembroke Dock. Cross the Haven by Cleddau Bridge. From Neyland the path follows the north shore through the town of Milford Haven (L) and across Sandy Haven on to the Dale Peninsular. The estuaries before this point can be crossed only at low tide: at other times an inland detour is necessary. A bus service from Dale to St Davids operates from Sunday to Friday in the summer. From Dale the path follows the coastline within sight of two off-shore islands—Skokholm and Skomer. It then rounds St Ann's Head and Wootlack Point and continues past the Stack Rocks up to Broad Haven where a special unit of the Countryside Commission has been set up to provide open-air lectures and walks.

From Broad Haven the path leads north around St Bride's Bay through the fishing village of Nolton Haven, along Newgale Sands, past Solva, and along the shoreline of Ramsey Sound just south of the town of St Davids, the birthplace of the patron saint of Wales. St Davids cathedral, situated in a shallow vale, was built in the twelfth century of purple stone, and has been a place of pilgrimage for centuries.

The route continues west around the head, past Ramsey Island where there is a colony of Atlantic seals, then turns north along Whitesands Bay to St David's Head (H) and the beginning of what I consider to be the best part of the path. For some forty to fifty miles the path follows dramatic cliffs and the remote hostels are a day's walk apart from each other.

From St David's Head the path goes north to Strumble Head by the Trevine and Pwll Deri Hostels; from there it continues east to Fishguard Bay after which the path climbs the rugged cliffs over Dinas Head to the resort of Newport (LH). North of Newport's sandy beach the path continues around Cemaes Head to its north

end at St Dogmaels on the river Teifi, passing Poppit Sands hostel
on the way.

WALKS IN SNOWDONIA

Snowdonia, 845 square miles of national park, is named after the
principal mountain in the park, Mount Snowdon, at 3560 feet the
highest and steepest mountain in England and Wales. The mountain
was, like most of its neighbours in Snowdonia, formed almost four
hundred million years ago of rocks which were the product of
Ordovician volcanoes; and through all those millenia the mountain
stood nameless until some brash Saxon invader saw it from the
distance, in summer, yet with snow still on its summit, and
commented "Snaudon", the snowy one, to distinguish it from its
sister mountains. The Welsh call the mountain Y Wyddfa Fawr
which means "the great burial place", referring, some say, to King
Arthur who is reputed to be buried on its summit.

Snowdon is only one of fourteen peaks in the park that are over
the three thousand foot level. There are centres for climbing at
Llanberis Pass, Nant Ffracon Pass, and Capel Curig. Cadair Idris,
at about three thousand feet, lies to the south and is for the
experienced climber only.

You can not go home without climbing Snowdon, and not just
because it's there. At the top, if the weather is clear, you could be
rewarded with a view over four counties; and if it is misty, which is
more likely to be the case, you may be rewarded by seeing a *glory*
around your *Brocken spectre*! A *Brocken spectre* was first
recorded in Brocken, Germany—hence the name; it is a shadow of
a climber cast upon the mist in a *cwm* or hollow. The shadow
looks very close and seems immense because it is an optical illusion
refracted on the mist. The *glory* is a coloured ring which is
sometimes visible around this spectre—but each climber can only
see his own *glory*.

Be very careful of the weather on the mountain because it
changes so quickly. You can start out in sunlight and be drenched
half an hour later by heavy mountain mist. Be sure to stay on the
paths, dress warmly and carry rain gear: you really can die of
exposure if you get lost on the mountain in a heavy mist.

There are two easy routes up to the summit and they correspond
with places already mentioned on the bike tour: the Snowdon
Ranger Track and the Llanberis Track.

Use Ordnance Survey maps 115 and 124 in the 1:50,000 Series for the following hikes and climbs in Snowdonia.

3. *Snowdon Ranger Track*

This is probably the oldest track up Snowdon; it starts at the back of the Snowdon Ranger Hostel and the ascent takes about two hours.

Outside the hostel take a few steps west on the road toward Caernarvon and then turn right through the white gate, cross the old railway line and make for the farm with the mill wheel. You are walking through private property here, so stay on the path. Turn right at the farm and follow the zig-zags of the path and the white arrows up the first five hundred feet. After this the path is easier, but sometimes tends to lose itself in boggy ground. Watch out for the sharp left after the second stream, and be sure to keep the wire fence on your right and the slopes of Moel Cynghorion on your left whilst heading straight to Bwlch Cwm Brwynog. When you get to the part where the path crosses close by the ridge of Bwlch Cwm Brwynog, it is worth climbing up the ridge to see the view north-west toward Llanberis. The path zig-zags steeply again, but is easy to follow in summer. It passes near the precipice of Clogwyn Du'r Arddu (the black cliff of the black height).

The Ranger track meets the track from Llanberis near Bwlch Glas, and from here it is only a ten minute walk to the summit.

The ascent is not as complicated as it may sound; once on the mountain it is quite easy to follow the path. You can buy a cheap guide at the hostel, and before setting off you should check with the warden about any recent deterioration or changes in the path.

4. *Llanberis Track*

This track starts on the main road almost opposite the Royal Victoria Hotel. If you are staying at the Llanberis Hostel, the path can be joined near Hebron Station by taking the road behind the hostel and crossing the foot of Cwm Brwynog. The path is signposted at the beginning and is so broad and well defined that no description is needed. Even eighty-year-olds have been known to make this ascent!

In summer there are no difficulties on the route; you should allow two and a half hours for the ascent. There are some superb views to be seen along the way—you even pass close to the head of Snowdon's most famous waterfall, Ceunant Mawr. As the two tracks meet at Bwlch Glas, you can make the climb from one hostel and descend to the other for the night. Be careful of the weather: even though the paths are well marked and easy to follow in good light, the mists make a world of difference up there and can roll in very quickly. As long as you stay on the track you should be safe even in bad weather.

There is also a narrow-gauge railway from Llanberis that makes the ascent and descent.

Snowdon has been to the British what Mount Everest has been to the world: ever since the eighteenth century when men of means followed the rough miner's tracks up the mountain, through the hey-day of ponies and guides and a B and B on top of the mountain for five shillings, until today when there are a dozen trails up the mountainside and a railway to boot—through all this time, Snowdon has remained a challenge and something to achieve. But there are days when the weather will not be good enough for the ascent, or when you just want to take it easy. If you are staying at the hostel you will have to be out during the day and there are lots of easy walks in Snowdonia. I give just one here from the Snowdon Ranger Hostel to Beddgelert, but there are many others.

5. *Snowdon Ranger Hostel to Beddgelert (8 miles)*

From the hostel follow the same directions given for the ascent of Snowdon as far as the railway line. Turn right to go eastwards along the disused line. The track meanders over pleasant countryside and crosses a stream that rushes under the trestle like a waterfall: an ideal place to stop for lunch. The track continues for about three miles on the north side of the A4085 and then comes out on the road about a mile beyond the tiny village of Rhyd-Ddu. From this point the railway line passes through private property and it is necessary to walk along the road for a bit until you approach a forest on your right, south of the main road, where you will find a path off the road which goes through the forest to Beddgelert, or, if you do not have a map of the region, you can stay on the road for two more miles into Beddgelert. The path continues on after Beddgelert: follow the little stream south and you will pass the grave of Gelert (from which the town takes its name). This is worth a short diversion off the path, even though I have heard the monument is a fake from the nineteenth century.

From the grave you can continue along the trail by the river for another mile to the south to a waterfall, which is more of a rapid than a waterfall but impressive nonetheless. Follow the trail back

into Beddgelert where you can catch a ramshackle old bus back to
Snowdon Ranger Hostel or to Caernarvon; it leaves at about forty
minute intervals, but check the timetable at the hostel before
leaving in the morning just to make sure.

WALKS IN THE BRECON BEACONS

The Brecon Beacons are a National Park. Pen-y-Fan is the
Snowdon of the Beacons, standing almost three thousand feet and
right in the centre of the park; but this park is not only mountains:
there are also vast stretches of open common land and pastoral
countryside, much of which is farmed.

Besides walking in the Beacons, there is also good rock climbing
on the limestone rocks in the south of the park. The main peaks of
the Beacons are sandstone and not good for climbing. This is good
pony-trekking country. A unique feature of the park are the vast
limestone caves which you can explore; although you can make
contact with a good caving club to find out how to navigate safely,
I would not recommend this sport to a beginner. Content yourself
instead with the caves open to the public: the Dan Yr Ogof and the
Cathedral Show Caves in the Tawe Valley.

Use Ordnance Survey maps in the 1:50,000 Series 160, 161, 170,
171 for walks and climbs in the Beacons.

6. *Canal Walk (33 miles)*
In addition to the hill walking in the Beacons Park, there is the
Monmouthshire and Brecon Canal, running from Pontypool in
the south to Brecon in the north, offering thirty-three miles of one
of the most beautiful canals in Britain. This canal was built, like
most of the two thousand miles of canal in Britain, in the
nineteenth century as a transportation route between industrial
and trading centres. You can rent boats for short trips along
various sections of the canal, or walk the whole way along the tow
path; and, as the canal was built to connect towns one with
another, you will find plenty of accommodation along the way.

7. *The Ascent of Pen-y-Fan (6 miles or 10 miles)*
The main climbing centre in the Beacons is at Libanus, just south-
west of Brecon, though Brecon itself is also a good starting point
for hikes. There are also several hostels in the park that can act as
centres for hikes around themselves.

There are many routes up Pen-y-Fan, and one of the easiest and best marked is the Gap Road. It follows an old Roman road and goes south up and over the Beacons.

From Brecon proceed south for about three miles on a minor road. Where the road ends walk up the stony land and through the gate on to the open hill which is National Trust property. Do not make for the ridge, but stay to the left, as the Roman road follows the east or left slope of Bryn-teg to reach the gap. From the gap ascend the east side of Cribbin and on up to Pen-y-Fan. Although the paths are fairly obvious, it is wise to carry a map. Always enquire about the paths locally before you set out.

From Pen-y-Fan it is possible to continue the journey to another hostel for the night, or to turn back and return to Brecon by the same route. The first part (the ascent) is six miles all together, but only three and a half miles of climbing, so allow about three to three and a half hours for this part.

To descend to another hostel, the Llwyn-y-Celyn, follow the path south-west from Pen-y-Fan to the left of Corn Du (unless you want to climb this peak also) which will take you straight down to a cairn at Bwlch Duwynt; from there you can follow a broad track on fairly level ground until you turn right (the path is marked) on to a path going downhill for half a mile and marked by white posts. (The routes to the right as you descend this portion will take you to a National Trust monument.) From here you descend obliquely right for quarter of a mile, cross the stream at the bottom by the stepping stones and pass through the gate into a lane which you follow on to the A470 road. Turn right, going north on the road for a short distance to the Storey Arms. These are complicated instructions, but only cover two miles. The route down may be wet and muddy.

From the telephone box by the Storey Arms another path leaves the A470 to the right and goes north following the fence quite closely along the foot of Y Gyrn; it will take you to the hostel at Llwyn-y-Celyn but you will have to ford the River Tarell; or you can just follow the A470 road north for the two miles to the hostel. The whole route is ten miles and you should allow ample daylight hours for finding the way.

8. *Cross Country in the Beacons (23 miles)*

You can do some cross-country walking in the Beacons from hostel to hostel. From the hostel at Llwyn-y-Celyn it is eleven miles to the hostel at Ystradfellte, in the waterfall country; and from

Ystradfellte another twelve miles to the hostel at Llanddeusant. The walk is via footpaths and minor roads. I have not done this particular walk, so I do not know how well marked the footpaths are once you are out in the field. It is best to check locally first, especially with the wardens at the hostels. The park information officer at Brecon, on Glamorgan Street, has many leaflets for sale with maps of walks in the Beacons. Be sure to use the Ordnance Survey maps in the 1:50,000 scale mentioned above.

NATURE TRAILS

Wales also has many short nature trails and forest trails, well marked and thematic, i.e. they introduce you to animals or trees or geological history with explanations on panels at points along the trails. There are about sixty trails, mostly in the north and far south of Wales, so look out for signs on the roadside. These trails are ideal for bikers who feel like a change.

SIX
Southern Ireland

And I shall have some peace there,
for peace comes dropping slow,
Dropping from the veils of the morning
to where the cricket sings.

W. B. YEATS: The Lake Isle of Innisfree

The Republic of Ireland, Eire or Southern Ireland is not part of Britain, neither politically nor culturally. This is another country, and it is surprising to find such striking differences from England only just across the narrow Irish Sea.

The English ruled Ireland from the twelfth century until the twentieth, yet Ireland still retains her own identity. Even the Irish currency is different. You can spend English pounds here but you cannot spend Irish pounds in Britain, so be sure to change your money in Ireland before leaving. There are not so many formalized institutions in Ireland as in England and everything seems to have a rough, unfinished nature to it—even the landscape. The Irish are much better about letting you camp out in their fields than are the English; but on maps of Ireland there are no red, dotted lines to follow to help you to find your way easily when hiking. The Irish are easy-going people, but their cities are by and large just trading centres and nothing to write home about as far as prettiness goes. In many ways Ireland is still pre-industrial, and that is both good and bad. It means that the countryside here is not yet greatly spoiled, but it also means that the people are often very poor. As one way of combating this poverty, large ugly industrial plants (such as Japanese aluminium plants) that cannot now be built anywhere else in the world because of waste and pollution, are built in Ireland. The Irish today are caught between the wish for an ecologically healthy nation and an economically functioning state. At present most young people are forced to leave the country to find a job.

Ireland has two thousand miles of coastline and nowhere can you be more than seventy miles from the sea. Topographically the country is one broad central plain surrounded almost completely by coastal highlands. There are the Wicklow Mountains, in the south-east, the mountains of Kerry in the south-west, and those of Donegal in the north-west. Ireland's sunniest months are May and June, though even then you can expect to get wet.

Ireland is a Catholic country and people still have large families, though there are many more pubs than churches or nurseries. You cannot turn round in an Irish city without bumping into a pub.

Ireland is a great fishing country, but licences are not cheap. Peat, cut from the ground in bricks, still heats many homes and now runs giant turbines in power plants. Look for the peat bogs all over the country—ditches cut into dark brown soil; and look for the gypsies who seem to line every lane, or be a gypsy yourself and rent a horse-drawn Romany caravan in County Cork to plod along the roads at a delicious snail's pace with your wooden home-on-wheels under you. Or stay at one of the hundreds of farmhouses all over the island; they offer a peaceful night's sleep and a hearty breakfast for a reasonable price.

If you like music, look out for signs advertising a real Irish musical get-together, called a *seisiun*. In the bike tours I will tell you where *seisiuns* are held, but places and times change over the years so you may want to write or visit the Traditional Music Society in Dublin for a current schedule. They can also advise you about classes given on traditional Irish music—you may even learn how to play the tin whistle while biking!

If you like good tweed, go to County Donegal where some of the best tweed in the world is woven. I hesitate to mention the over-rated Irish sweater— in recent years the quality has been going down and the price up, but they are for sale everywhere and they are warm.

There are regions of Ireland which I think are over-rated, but which attract many people. The South-West is the most obvious example, counties Cork and Kerry. In the summer there are thousands of tourists in these two counties for no other reason than reputation; while comparably scenic areas to the north remain virtually unvisited.

Ireland, like Wales and Scotland, has strong Celtic origins: origins both of culture and language. The Irish, or Gaelic language is the oldest written vernacular in Europe, and Ireland was a Gaelic speaking country until the middle of the last century. There are areas, especially in the West, where Gaelic is still heard in everyday speech. The areas where Gaelic is spoken are called *Gaeltacht* districts. Gaelic is used on road and street signs together with English, and public transport destinations are shown in both languages. The following short glossary may help you and be of interest when trying to understand the meanings of place names:

ar(d): a high place
ath: ford
bally: townland
bag: small
bawn: a fortified enclosure
    attached to a castle
caher: a stone fort
carrig: rock
cashel: a stone fort
derg: red
derry, dare: oak tree or wood
drum: ridge, hillock
dun: a fort
feis: assembly, Gaelic festival
feis ceoil: music festival
fert: grave
fleadh ceoil: festival of
    ballad singing and
    traditional music

Gaeltacht: district where Irish is
    spoken as the vernacular
Inch, innis: island, river meadow
ken: head
kil: church, cell
knock: hill
lis: an earthen fort
lough: lake
more: great
oughter: upper
owen, avon: river
sept: clan
skerry: rock
slieve: mountain
teampall: church
tholsel: town hall
tober, tubber: well
tra: beach
tully: hillock

There are several ways to get to and depart from Ireland, but my favourite is by sea. There are airports, however, near Dublin in the east and at Shannon near Limerick in the west.

If you go by sea you will be travelling on English ferries and your bike will cost half the adult second-class passage. The crossing from Wales to Ireland takes from three to five hours. You can sail from either Fishguard in South Wales to land at Rosslare, some 120 miles south of Dublin, or from Holyhead in North Wales to land at Dublin's port of Dun Laoghaire (pronounced Dun Leary).

Ireland is a good biking country—fairly flat and easy-going with little heavy traffic once you are thirty to fifty miles out of Dublin. Roads in Ireland have a different numbering system from that in England. "T" roads are trunk roads or main roads; "N" means a national route and is the same size as a T road, the only difference being that N roads link up cross-country. However, sometimes the entire N road system is made up of many stretches of T roads (lettered and numbered so only in a local area) and thus the same road may be a T and an N at the same time, and in this case, the T is usually in parentheses on the routes or on the maps. "L" means a link road and is like the B roads of England. Other smaller routes that are unlettered and un-numbered I refer to as minor roads and give the destination as a means of identification. As the N and T roads carry less traffic than the main roads in England, many of the bike routes use major roads.

Ireland is a flat country but prevailing winds along the coast can make biking hard work. The wind usually comes from the south-west but it changes around the coast where it always seems to blow in from the sea.

I provide five tours for bikers in Ireland, covering something like a thousand miles, plus an alternate route from Rosslare. This is probably a much greater distance than you will want to cover. I think the two best parts of Ireland are the Wicklows and Donegal, with the counties of Galway and Clare coming a close third. The bike routes start in the Wicklows, to the south of Dublin, and proceed more or less clockwise around the island. You can of course shorten the length of the entire circuit very easily by taking trains between major touring areas. Also do not forget that buses sometimes carry bikes in Ireland.

Ireland is a much better biking country than a hiking country because there is no well organized public footpath system in Ireland, and there are none of the convenient long distance footpaths that exist in Britain. Rights of way are not so well defined in Ireland, and the hiker can strike off across many miles of open land with only compass and map as guides. Ireland has many little-used minor roads that can be used by the hiker. In addition, there are several mountain climbing and hill walking centres, usually based around the youth hostels. You can generally get information about mountain paths at the hostels.

I supply eight hiking and climbing paths for Ireland, some are in mountainous and hilly country, others in the flat-lands. Some use pathways, others use minor roads and canal tow-paths. They are based around hostels and many routes lead from hostel to hostel over mountains or hills. Do not be afraid to strike off on your own on the paths and minor roads. Just be sure that you have a good supply of Irish Ordnance Survey maps in the one-inch series and some knowledge of how to find the way.

Hitch-hiking is very easy in Ireland, I have even known people to stop for a biker whose bike has broken down, and transport bike and rider into the next village for repairs.

BIKING

WHAT TO DO IF YOU LAND AT ROSSLARE

There are three alternatives to choose from:

Rosslare to Dublin (120 miles)

The simplest thing, if you want to see Dublin first and begin the biking tours in order, is to take the train or bus up to Dublin, but this will not be cheap; or you could bike all the way. It will cost a lot in money or in time and energy, whichever you prefer.

Alternatively you could join up with the first bike tour at Kilkenny. By doing this you would miss the Wicklows, but you could do a couple of days of touring from Dublin into the Wicklows later on.

Rosslare to Kilkenny (60 miles)

Take a minor road south-west from Rosslare for Killinick and on to the T8 going north through Wexford (CL) the capital of County Wexford and at once a busy industrial town and lovely ancient city with narrow, winding streets.

Take the T12 west from Wexford to New Ross (L), another town of medieval appearance. From here go north on the T20 through Thomastown in the fine valley of the River Nore; continue north into Kilkenny and join the first bike tour of Ireland there.

Rosslare to Glendalough (75 miles)

This is a compromise between the first two options and is the one I recommend. You will still visit Dublin at the end of the journey, but you see some of the Wicklows while you are still fresh to Ireland.

On this route you go to Wexford from Rosslare (see the previous route), then proceed north on the L29 and bear right on to the L30 through Curracloe (CL). At Blackwater turn on to a minor road going north through Ford. The next part part of the route is near good, long stretches of open beach. Continue through Courtown

(LC), a popular resort on the seaside, and past the Hill of Tara (not *the* Hill of Tara) and on to the T7 going north at Scarnagh cross roads. Continue through Arklow (LC), another very popular seaside resort, at the mouth of the Avoca River.

From here you stay on the T7 north-west along the Vale of Avoca, which in late spring explodes with white blossoms against the green foliage. In this vale, you will pass through the lovely villages of Woodenbridge (L), which was the heart of a goldrush in 1796, and Avoca (L). You are now in real Wicklow country, yet different from the Wicklow mountains to be seen further to the west.

From Avoca continue north past the Meeting of the Waters, where two rivers, the Avonmore and the Avonberg come together. As the tour guides would tell you over the microphones on the coaches, this is a place of "sylvan beauty". North of here is Rathdrum (L), another lovely valley town, this time on the Avonmore River. At Rathdrum follow the T61 north-west along the banks of the Avonmore River to Laragh, and then on to the L107 by a left turn to Glendalough (H), where you join the bike tour of the Wicklows in the early stages of its course. (See the following bike tour.)

THE WICKLOWS and TIPPERARY
(165 miles)

The bike routes in The Wicklows and Tipperary are covered by map 4 in the Irish Ordnance Survey Quarter-Inch Series, and by maps 16, 18, 19 and 23 in the Half-Inch series.

The Wicklows (60 miles)

From Dublin take the T43 a few miles south out of the city to the village of Dundrum, then take minor roads south to the L93 where you turn left, east, for one mile until you come to another minor road to the right, south, for Glencullen and Enniskerry (LH). Turn right on this road into Enniskerry, a place praised as one of the prettiest villages in Ireland (see under *Hiking*). Near Enniskerry is Powerscourt Demesne, one of the loveliest homes in Ireland and open to the public. From Enniskerry take a minor road west for the Glencree Hostel and then turn left, south, on the L94 road which takes you into the heart of the Wicklow Mountains. There is fine mountain, woodland and moorland scenery in store for you here, and wooded glens that are almost too much. This area used to be the rebel stronghold of the Irish, until the English built good roads into its heart.

Continue south on the L94 to Sally Gap where you turn right, north-west, on the L161 for Kibride where you turn left, south, on a minor road for Blessington (LH), a pleasant little village of one long street, situated by a reservoir which serves as Dublin's water supply. From Blessington go south by minor roads for a few miles to the L107 at the Wicklow Gap (H) and turn left, south-east, passing through Glendalough (H), an area of wild scenic beauty where you can see the ruins of a famous monastery, founded by St Keven in the seventh century and renowned throughout Europe in its day as a centre of learning.

The existence of monasteries in Ireland during the Dark Ages is significant in relation to the historical figure of King Arthur. Arthur is thought by historians to be important because he gave the native Britains a generation of safety from the onslaught of the barbaric Saxons and Angles. This gave the fledgling monastic movement in England and Ireland time to consolidate as centres for the preservation of learning. Indeed, Arthur and Celts like him prevented the invaders from even reaching Ireland, which was not invaded until the twelfth century, and then by the Normans. After the fall of the Roman Empire classical learning was lost save in monasteries such as Glendalough and similar places all over Europe where Western Civilization weathered the storm of the Dark Ages. Ireland was for a time the main centre of learning in the Western world.

The monasteries usually have a church and cloister and kitchens and possibly also a tall, round tower, which it is thought would have been used as a watch-tower and fort.

Continue south-east into Laragh and then on to a minor road going south for about five miles until you reach a turning to the right, north-west, up the beautiful Glenmalur. Continue past the hostel in the glen, over Table Mountain, past the Ballinclea Hostel and then into Donard on another minor road going north-west.

This completes the biking tour of the Wicklows and we now move on towards Kilkenny and into Tipperary County. (See under *Hiking* for a walk in the Wicklows.)

Donard to Kilkenny (50 miles)

This is a connecting route. There is a station to the north of Donard at Nass where you can catch a train to Kilkenny, also a bus

The Wicklows and Tipperary

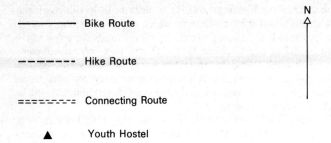

Bike Route

Hike Route

Connecting Route

▲ Youth Hostel

N

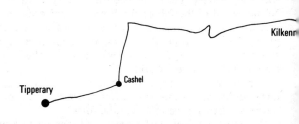

Kilkenn

Cashel

Tipperary

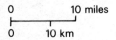

0   10 miles

0   10 km

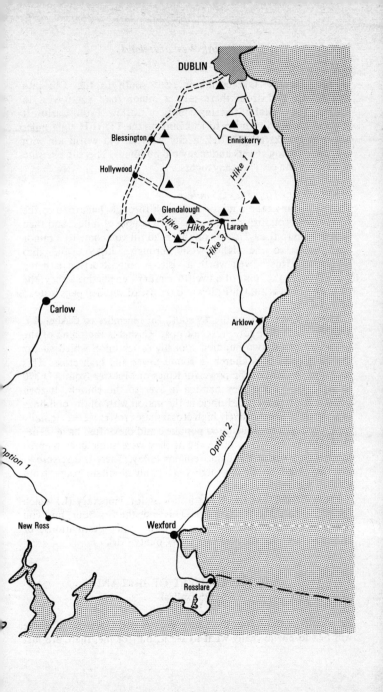

if you do not wish to bike.

From Donard take a minor road south to the T42 into Baltinglass, and from there take a minor road south-west to Carlow, the capital of the tiny county of Carlow. From Carlow it is about twenty-five miles to Kilkenny on the T51 (LH eight miles north at Foulksrath Castle), a city with an old world air with narrow, winding streets and many old buildings. There is a *seisiun* at Kytelers Inn on Thursday nights.

Kilkenny to Tipperary (55 miles)

From Kilkenny take a minor road west through Tullaroan to the L153 where you turn right, north, for a couple of miles, and then turn left on to the L27; stay on this road till you come to a minor road going to the right, west, through Littleton and into Holycross. This is well worth a visit. A reconstruction is being carried out in the ruins of a twelfth century Benedictine abbey; the reconstruction is authentic down to the use of wooden pegs instead of metal nails.

From Holycross take the T9 south for ten miles to Cashel (L), another place that you must not miss. Cashel is the name of the town and of the two hundred foot high rock upon which sit the dramatic ruins of a church, a round tower and high cross. This rock was the seat of the powerful Kings of Munster from AD 370 to AD 1101, when they handed it over to the church. It then became the strongest bishopric in the nation with all the buildings to go with it. See the lovely high cross; these crosses were originally meant to teach the unlettered populace and they often have scenes from the Bible carved upon them; they were sometimes painted though no trace of the paint remains today. There is a *seisiun* at the City Hall on Friday nights. (For an alternate route from Cashel, see the next tour.)

From Cashel take the N74 south-west for Tipperary (L) which means in Irish, the Well of Ara. This ends the first tour, and you can either get a train at Tipperary for other destinations, or continue south for the next tour into County Cork.

THE SOUTH-WEST OF IRELAND
(255 miles)

Personally, I think that the South-West is often over-rated; there will be those who really want to see it, but for me, there are just too many tourists in the summer to make the area attractive.

The route I give of 255 miles could easily be extended to over three hundred miles if you include the alternate route around the Dingle Peninsula, which is actually one of the best parts of the South-West. Aside from that you will find many of the places most lauded in tourist books about Ireland: Blarney Castle, the Ring of Kerry and the Lakes of Killarney.

The bike routes in The South-West of Ireland are covered by map 5 in the Irish Ordnance Survey Quarter-Inch Series, and by maps 17, 18, 20, 21, 22 and 24 in the Half-Inch Series.

Tipperary to Cork (55 miles)

From Tipperary, if you decide to bike to Cork, take the L119 south-west out of the town through Galbally and on to the T50 for Mitchelstown (L), a busy dairy centre—try Mitchelstown cheddar cheese. Ten miles east of the town up the T6 there are over a mile of underground limestone caverns with stalactite and stalagmite phantasmagoria.

You may want to stop the last tour at Cashel as suggested above, and continue south from there on the T9 to Caher instead of going to Tipperary. In this way you could approach the Mitchelstown Caves from the east and avoid backtracking. Caher (L) is a lovely and bustling little town with a fine old castle. Proceed from here on T6 to Mitchelstown.

From Mitchelstown you take the T6 south for Fermoy (L), a good fishing centre on the banks of the Blackwater River. If planning to stop overnight in the area I advise staying at Mrs Young's beautiful old farmhouse in Kilworth, three miles north of Fermoy. She serves delicious high teas and the farm is set in the midst of fine bucolic scenery. From Fermoy go west on the T30 for Ballyhooly and then south from there on a minor road for the L188 leading south into Cork City (CLH). This is a sprawling port and Ireland's third largest city. It is also a university town and there are plenty of churches and libraries. Take a walk on the Grand Parade and St Patrick's Street; and try the Oyster Bar for good food, though a trifle on the expensive side. There are also some second-hand book shops, and a *seisiun* at the Country Club Hotel on Wednesday nights. Cork is usually full to the brim with visitors in the summer months so make reservations for accommodation from some other tourist office in Ireland before you arrive.

Cork to Glengariff (75 miles)

From Cork it is only five miles to Blarney Castle and village (L) via the L69 north-west through Killens Cross. If you have got as far as this you really cannot go home without going to the castle and giving the old stone a kiss—a kiss which is supposed to grant you eloquence. From Blarney take the L69 west to a minor road half a mile away and across the L9 continuing on the same minor road to meet the T29 where you turn right, west. This road travels between Cork and the coast via the beautiful Lee Valley, through Dripsey and Coachford and into Macroom (L), a nice little market town with a castle—try the River Inn Pub, it has Country and Western music and chips late at night.

From Macroom follow the T64 through Inchigeelagh (L), supposedly a favourite haunt of artists; and through Ballingeary (H) where there is a Gaelic school in the summer and a good climbing centre. From here you go over the difficult but lovely Pass of Keimaneigh, which is an uphill walk of one and a half miles, but a great downhill run for several miles through isolated country. As you get farther away from Dublin, you will notice that the distance between individual houses increases: in this part of the south-west, and later in the far north-west you will see about the largest social distance in Europe in the midst of one of the most popular touring areas in Ireland.

Continue into Ballylickey and then into Glengariff (LC) which is a lovely little village strewn along the main road and up the hills around Bantry Bay, but, for its size, very over-crowded in summer.

Glengariff to Kenmare (35 miles)

From Glengariff go south-west on the L61 for eleven miles to Adrigole and then turn right, north, on to a minor road to go over the Healy Pass, past the hostel at Glanmore Lake (see under *Hiking*), to Lauragh where you take the L62 north-east for Kenmare (L). This is a tourist town on the Kenmare River and is the southern centre for tours of the fabled Ring of Kerry.

Ring of Kerry (75 miles)

The Ring of Kerry is one of those guide-book musts but not one of my favourite areas. There are pretty and even spectacular parts on this tour around the Kerry peninsula; but the biking is difficult with many long climbs and stiff winds to fight. Coupled with this is the fact that the road around the Ring of Kerry is a major one, though not very wide, and is one of the busiest stretches of road in all Ireland.

Take the T66 south-west from Kenmare to Sneem. The River Sneem is good for trout and salmon fishing. From here it is twenty-one miles to Waterville, another fishing centre and European watering-place. Charlie Chaplin spent summers here for many years. Ballinskelligs (CH) is a Gaelic speaking fishing village not far to the west. There is a *seisiun* at Ostlann Rinn Rua on Wednesday nights. You can rent a boat from Ballinskelligs and go out to the Skellig Rocks off the mainland where there used to be a monastic settlement. The monks settled on an island in the hope of finding some protection from raiders.

From Ballinskelligs it is ten miles north on the T66 to Cahersiveen (LH on Valencia Island—take the ferry at Valencia Harbour). Still on the T66 but eighteen miles farther on is Glenbeigh (L), a good fishing and walking centre. From Glenbeigh it is eight miles to Killorglin (LH seven miles away on the Killarney road—see under *Hiking*) and the end of the Ring of Kerry.

Killarney is thirteen miles from Killorglin. It is or was a pretty little town, but in the high season it is flooded with people going to see the lakes, the Ring of Kerry, and Muckross Abbey and Ross Castle to the south.

Dingle Peninsula (90 miles)

I include this tour as an alternative to the Ring of Kerry. It does not have the spectacular scenery of the Ring, but the Dingle Peninsula has its own charm. If you saw the film, *Ryan's Daughter* you will know what to expect for it was filmed on the Dingle Peninsula. This area is more traditional and less touristy than most other parts of the south-west, and also has fine coastal scenery; it is more barren, more wild and primitive than the Ring. It is a Gaeltacht area.

With alternate routes this peninsula can give you a ninety mile journey. You go from Killorglin north on the N70 to Castlemaine where you turn left, travelling west on the L103 on to the peninsula via Inch (L), then on to the T68 to Dingle (L), which is a centre for the ascent of the Brandon Mountains.

From Dingle you can do a thirty mile round trip out to the farthest reaches of the peninsular, via a minor road west through Ventyr and past the famous archaeological remains called the Fahan Group. This consists of many standing stones with a writing system, called "Ogham" writing, inscribed in lines along their

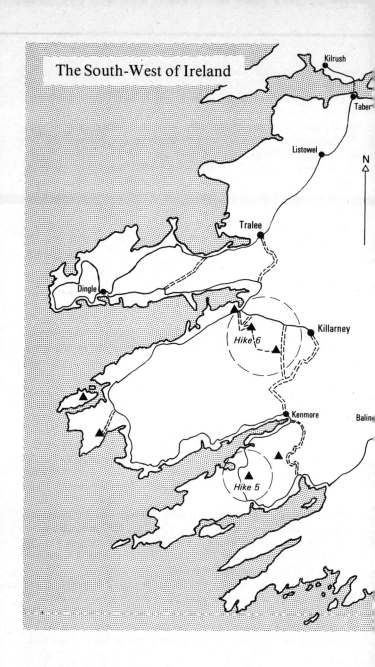

The South-West of Ireland

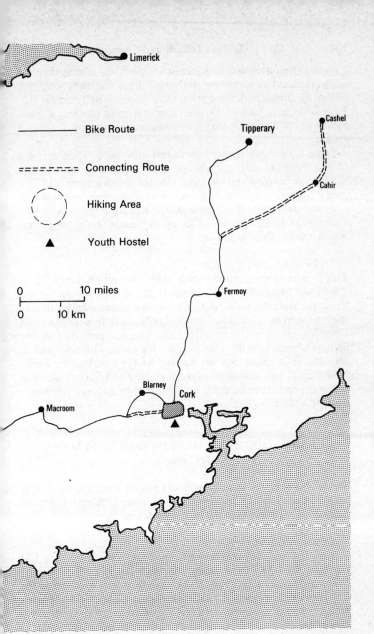

Limerick

Tipperary

Cashel

Cahir

———— Bike Route

======= Connecting Route

⌒ Hiking Area

▲ Youth Hostel

0   10 miles
0   10 km

Fermoy

Blarney

Cork

Macroom

▲

corners. There are also many prehistoric burial sites in the shape of cairns (hillocks of stone over the burial). Continue on through the village of Dunquin (L) and from there north to Ballyferriter (L), Ballydavid, and back to Dingle. This route will give you a good survey of the tip on the Dingle Peninsular in the remote Gaeltacht region.

From Dingle you proceed north-east on a minor road over the Conair Pass (which can be rough going), and loop left off that road on to another minor road through Castlegregory (LC), a pretty village but with no castle remaining; and then back down to the road going into Tralee, on which you turn right, east, into Tralee (L), the chief town of Kerry and home of the songwriter who wrote the *Rose of Tralee*.

Tralee to Kilrush (35 miles)

This is a connecting route which takes you into County Clare. Take the T68 north through Listowell (L) to the ferry at Tarber. Cross the river Shannon to the County Clare side where you take the N67 west into Kilrush. Tarber is only thirty-five miles east of Limerick, which is fifteen miles from Shannon airport. I do not include Limerick on this tour as it is a big town, with not much to see, and it is rather out of the way of the best touring areas. However, if you choose to make a journey to Limerick you can rejoin the main tour by going north-west through Ennis just below the Cliffs of Moher.

CLARE, THE ARAN ISLANDS and CONNEMARA
(215 miles)

The bike routes in Clare, Connemara and on Aran are covered by map 3 in the Irish Ordnance Survey Quarter-Inch Series, and by maps 10, 11, 14 and 17 in the Half-Inch Series.

Kilrush to Galway (100 miles)

Kilrush (LC) is a big marketing town. From Kilrush take the L54 north to join the T69. Continue through the villages of Quilty, Miltown Malbay (L), Lehinch (L); then turn left, west, on to the L54 through Liscannor (L) and past the dramatic Cliffs of Moher which rise some seven hundred feet out of the ocean and stretch for five miles.

Continue north through the spa of Lisdoonvarna (L), on to the

T69 for two miles and then on minor roads towards Formayle in the fifty square mile region known as the Burren. Together with the Cliffs of Moher, this is the most amazing part of a journey through Clare. The Burren is a limestone desert, the rock being covered with soil in only a few spots where quite exotic flowers bloom. This area is a speleologist's delight with limestone caves abounding.

Follow minor roads south-east then join the T69 which you follow north through Ballyvaghan (L), through the village of Burren, near the hostel at Kinvarra Bay, and into the town of Kinvarra (L) where there are nightly feasts at Dongory Castle. Ask at the local tourist board about these feasts, they are not cheap but can be a lot of fun in an old castle, lit only by candlelight, with minstrels and serving wenches. Continue north from here on the T69 to Kilcolgan (L).

There is an alternate route that adds about fifteen miles on to the total mileage of the tour. The detour leaves the main route at the village of Burren and rejoins it at Kilcolgan; it includes Thor Ballylee, the summer residence of the poet W. B. Yeats, which is now a sort of Yeats Museum. Yeats bought the sixteenth century tower-house for thirty-five pounds in 1917 and wrote the poems, *The Tower* and *The Winding Stair* here. Follow the minor road for Gort to the right off the T69 just three miles out of the village of Burren. At Gort (L) go north-east on the L11 and Thor Ballylee is four miles up this road. Past the tower is a minor road going off to the left, west, that joins the T11 at Ardrahan, then north-east of this point in the T11 you come into Kilcolgan and rejoin the main route.

Continue on north on the T11 to join the T4, west, into Galway (LC), one of the prettiest of Irish towns. Salthill, its seaside, honky-tonk resort is to be avoided unless you enjoy crowds of sunburned tourists smelling of baby oil and chips. August is race month and many people, mostly Irish, flock here to bet on the horses. Lodgings are at a premium and the town goes wild during the races.

Aran Islands (30 miles)

Galway is the gateway to the fabulous Aran Islands and to Connemara. First the islands. They lie a few hours of rough sea away from the mainland and are reached by boat from Galway harbour. These islands are still fairly remote and very desolate and dramatic—though do not expect the drama that the playwright

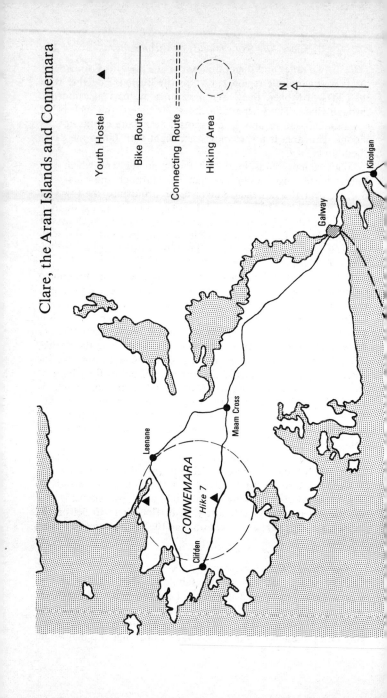

Clare, the Aran Islands and Connemara

▲ Youth Hostel

—— Bike Route

===== Connecting Route

⊙ Hiking Area

← N

Kilcolgan

Galway

Maam Cross

Leenane

Clifden

CONNEMARA
Hike 7

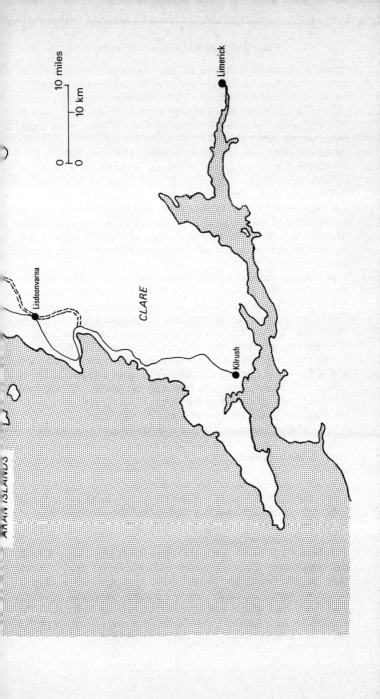

Synge wrote of in *Riders to the Sea*. Gone are the days of the rugged fishermen braving the waters of the treacherous Atlantic in their rough-hewn curraghs. Today the fishermen meet the boats to escort the tourists to their lodgings in horse-drawn traps; and do not expect the islanders to wear home-made traditional dress, Woolworths now clothe the populace. The tourist's loss is the islander's gain; well, sometimes anyway. The Aran Islands, bare limestone outcroppings in the ocean, still retain a sense of differentness.

There are three islands in the Aran group, and by boat from Galway you will land at Kilronan (LC) on Inishmore. There are no street lights on the island as most electricity is home-generated. There is a pub in Kilronan that is an old thatched-roof, dirt-floored cottage, where old salts sit around and swap sea stories in Gaelic.

Mini-bikes can be rented on the island and there is little motorized traffic on the few roads. It is perfect walking or biking country. Do not be put off if the tourist office in Galway city says there is no accommodation on Aran. The islanders have their own little tourist board set up in a trailer by the dock and there is plenty of lodging on the island, plus camping sites just outside Kilronan.

The main road on the island runs east/west between Kilronan and Kilmurvy (L), about six miles away. Dun Aengus, near the village of Kilmurvy, is a huge Iron Age fort (about two thousand years old) perched high over the ocean. From the fort you can see the Cliffs of Moher across the waters on the mainland. The fort was circular at one time, but one side has slipped into the sea, so that now you feel like a bird perched up there, so high and so far away from everything.

Connemara: Galway to Leenaun (80 miles)

Connemara is the western part of the county of Galway. It has superb mountain and peat bog scenery and the area is dominated by the mountains known as the Twelve Bens. It is very wild and very Irish—another Gaeltacht region.

Take the T71 north through Oughterard (L) by Lough Corrib and then west to Maam Cross (twenty-seven miles). Here you can take an alternate route on the L100 to Leenaun via Joyce's Country which is really lovely, rugged moorland, a very traditional area where you may not be able to understand the English spoken, let alone the Gaelic. However, if you take this route you will miss most of the heart of Connemara.

The main route continues west from Maam Cross on the T71 through the town of Recess—a choice beauty spot—and past the hostel of Ben Lettery (see under *Hiking*) at the foot of the Twelve Bens. From here the route continues on to Clifden (L) on the same road. Clifden is a Victorian seaside resort in an almost alpine setting. From Clifden it is another twenty-one miles, through beautiful Connemara scenery, along the T71 to Leenaun. I cannot say much about Leenaun because the only day I was there it was raining like the beginning of the Flood and we stopped only long enough to warm up in the pub over a shot of Irish whisky. North of Leenaun the route goes into County Mayo and the next touring area.

THE NORTHWEST PASSAGE and COUNTY DONEGAL
(350 miles)

You can reduce the length of this route by 150 miles by taking public transport to Donegal town and beginning your biking there, completing a circular route of County Donegal and then biking back down to Sligo town. When you read through this tour you will see how much you may need to backtrack. But do not miss Donegal—a rugged and grand area with good isolated beaches; it is hard biking country though and the distances are long.

The bike routes in the North-West and County Donegal are covered by maps 1 and 3 in the Irish Ordnance Survey Quarter-Inch Series and by maps 1, 3, 7 and 11 in the Half-Inch Series.

Leenaun to Sligo (90 miles)

This connecting route can be avoided by taking a bus from Leenaun or by biking to Westport twenty miles north on the T71 where you can catch a train. The following route takes you through Counties Mayo and Sligo, which are pretty areas, but not very different from what you may already have seen. (You can make a detour off the route to Achill Island. This would be a forty-mile round-trip.)

Take the T71 north through Westport (L), a very pretty fishing centre, and north-east through Castlebar on the T39, and then on to the T40 into Swinford (L), a quiet market town. From Swinford take a minor road north through Aclare into County Sligo, on to the T3 at Collooney and north into Sligo town (L). Sligo is a fairly large town, but rather nondescript.

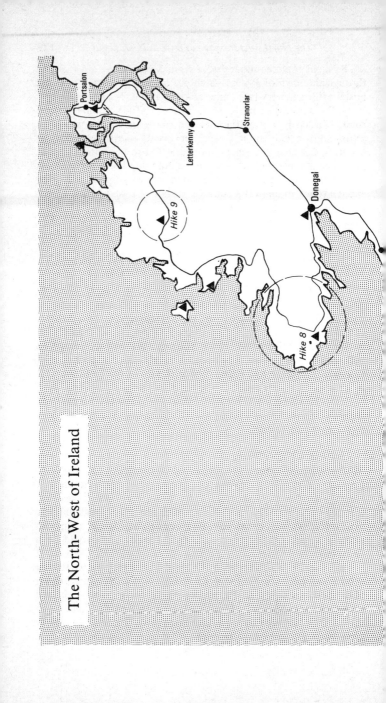

The North-West of Ireland

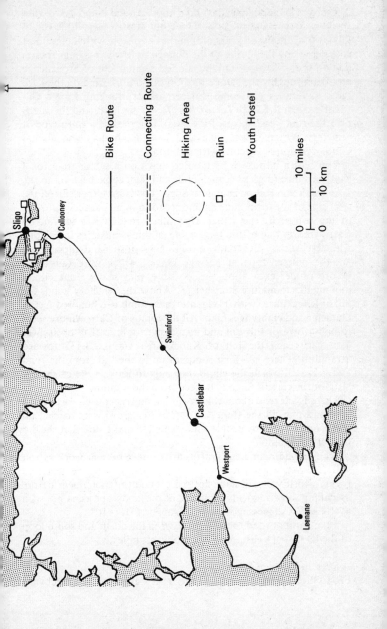

Bike Route

Connecting Route

Hiking Area

Ruin □

Youth Hostel ▲

Sligo
Collooney
Swinford
Castlebar
Westport
Leenane

0   10 miles
0   10 km

There is a good one day bike tour around Sligo town that includes archaeological sites. These are mostly Megalithic tombs (about four thousand years old) in the cairn style with a mound of rocks covering the burial, or the dolmen style where a huge rock is laid on top of several standing stones, reminiscent of Stonehenge and from roughly the same time. Go east out of Sligo on the L16. After five miles you come to Deerpark overlooking Lough Gill (Yeat's poem the *Lake Isle of Innisfree* is set here, and the isle is near the south-east shore of the lake). Deerpark is a cairn type of cemetery. When it was excavated in 1884, human and animal bones were found together with flint tools.

You return into town by looping down on a minor road for a short distance to go by Lough Gill, and then come back on to the L16 which you follow back into Sligo. To visit another site on the west side of the town, take a minor road running parallel with, but to the south of, the L132. The minor road will lead you by Carrowmore, one of the largest Megalithic cemeteries in Europe with at least sixty-five tombs sprouting out of the landscape. There are the dolmen type of passage graves, which were ransacked before proper excavation was possible, plus many stone circles looking like miniature Stonehenges. Above the cemetery stands the hill of Knocknarea with its gigantic cairn tomb two hundred feet in diameter and eighty feet high. All the tombs of Carrowmore seem to point towards this hill and its massive tomb as if in obeisance. You can reach the hill of Knocknarea via the L132 toward Strandhill. There is a long footpath up to the hill from the road and it is well worth the climb, not only to look at the cairn, but also for the view of Sligo to be seen from the summit.

There is a legend about this cairn that an Irish queen was buried here and that all the stones on top of her grave were carried up there, one by one, by people who wanted to make sure that she did not get out again.

Many modern amateur graffiti artists have been at work as you will discover when you reach the top. Below you the scattered rocks, which you will have noticed around the monument before ascending, now suddenly jump out of the landscape as names such as "Nigel" and messages such as "Amanda Does It".

Take a minor road to the left, between the north and south loop of the L132, back east into Sligo, about six miles.

Sligo to Donegal (45 miles)

From Sligo go north on the T18 to Yeat's grave at the churchyard of Drumcliff, under the unusual promontory of Benbulben. Continue north on the T18 into County Donegal, through the busy resort of Bundoran (CL), where there is a *seisiun* on Wednesday nights at the Shane House Hotel, and through the market and industrial town of Ballyshannon. Stay on the same road north through the village of Ballintra to Donegal town (LH), a sprightly robust place of a few thousand people.

Donegal to Mount Erigal (70 miles)

Donegal is the gateway to my favourite Irish county. County Donegal is the most northerly county in the Republic of Ireland, it has the best scenery and a generally unspoiled air: there are mountains, lakes, glens and empty beaches, and friendly people who have not yet been soured by the deluge of visitors that have descended upon Ireland in recent years.

From Donegal town go west on the T72 through the pleasant fishing village of Killybegs (L) where you can buy some of the best woollen socks in the world at any of the fishing or hardware stores. The fishermen wear these sturdy socks which are knitted from wool of many variegated colours and are superbly warm. Try also the caraway cake at the local bakery. Continue on the T72 through Kilian, a centre for the fine Donegal tweed, and on into Carrick (LH), where you must spare some time to see the magnificent cliffs at Slieve League and perhaps even climb the mountain (see under *Hiking*).

Take a minor road north and east from Carrick for Ardara, another tweed centre; continue on another minor road from there through Maas and then on to the T72 for twelve miles to Dunglow (H) at nearby Crohy Head. Dunglow leads into the Rosses (from the Irish words *Na Rosa* meaning "headlands") which are sixty thousand acres of rock-strewn land cut through by rivers and lakes. Take the L130 north to Gweedore, which is on the fringe of the so-called Bloody Foreland—the name derives from the colour the land assumes under the sun. From Gweedore go east on the L130 for a few miles and then on to the L82 to the hostel at Mount Erigal (see under *Hiking*).

Mount Erigal to Letterkenny (80 miles)

Continue east on the L82 and then turn left, north, on to minor roads for Creeslough on the T72. From here continue on the T72 through Carrickart (hostel nearby at Tra Na Rosann), and south to Milford (L). Take the L78 north to Carrowkeel (C) and then on to minor roads north to the Fanad Peninsula, through Roasnakil and on up north to Fanad Head (L) with its cliffs. Loop back down south on minor roads through Doagh Beg and Portsalon (L), the biggest tourist centre of the peninsula. Take the L78 south from Portsalon for a mile until you can turn left on to a minor road south-east for the hostel at Bunnaton on Lough Swilly. From Bunnaton continue south on minor roads back on to the L77, through the resort of Rathmullan (L) and Rathmelton, a fishing centre. It is eight miles on the T72 from there to Letterkenny (L), the chief town of Donegal.

Letterkenny to Sligo (75 miles)

Take the T59 south out of Letterkenny through Stranolar (L), where the T59 becomes the T18. Go south through Ballybofey and over the Barnesmore Gap to Donegal town. From here retrace your original route back to Sligo.

THE IRISH MIDLANDS to THE BOYNE VALLEY
(200 miles)

This tour takes you cross-country on a connecting route to an archaeological and historical tour in the Boyne Valley just north of Dublin. (The connecting route to the Boyne Valley is more functional than attractive, so you may prefer to take the train from Sligo.)

The bike routes in The Midlands and the Boyne Valley are covered by maps 1, 2 and 4 in the Irish Ordnance Survey Quarter-Inch Series, and by maps 7, 12 and 13 in the Half-Inch Series.

Sligo to Kells, (105 miles)

Take the N4 for fifty-seven miles to Longford. You will pass through Boyle (L) and Carrick-on-Shannon (L), a pretty little town on the River Shannon, a good fishing centre with a *seisiun* on Friday nights at the Bush Hotel. From there it is twenty-three miles to Longford (L), a hurly-burly, bustling market town, the centre of the Irish Midlands.

Take the T15 from Longford east through Granard, then the T24 for five miles until you meet the intersection with the T10 which you take south to Finnea. From Finnea continue on backroads: a minor road south-east for about twelve miles to the L3 into Crossakiel, and then the L142 east to Kells (L).

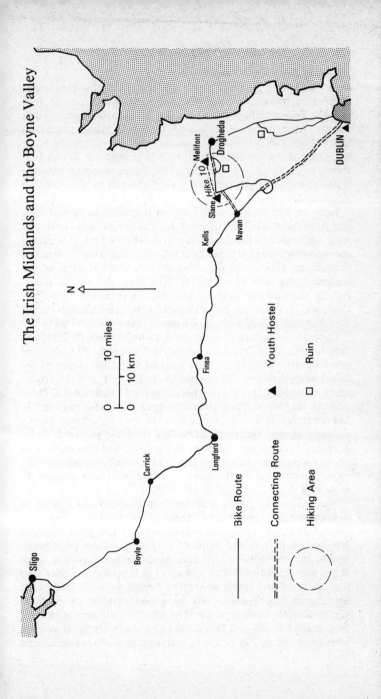

The Irish Midlands and the Boyne Valley

N

10 miles
10 km
0

Sligo
Boyle
Carrick
Longford
Finea
Kells
Navan
Slane
Hike 10
Melifont
Drogheda
DUBLIN

Bike Route
Connecting Route
Hiking Area
▲ Youth Hostel
□ Ruin

Kells to Drogheda (55 miles)

Kells used to be a monastic centre, and it was here that the famous illuminated manuscript, the Book of Kells (which can be seen today at Trinity College Library in Dublin), was made in the ninth century. At the main church in Kells there is an assortment of old high crosses with scenes carved on them in low relief. Kells is the beginning of the last "thematic" tour in Ireland but ironically it should be the first, for here in the Boyne Valley, along the pleasant banks of this fine river, much of the early history of Ireland lies in the green fields.

Take the T35 south-east into Navan (L), itself an ancient city, and from there take the T35 south for about eight miles until you see a minor road to the right going to the Hill of Tara. About two miles down this road is the ancient hill of the high kings of Ireland, in use from about 2000 BC onwards. Not much remains of the ancient dining hall or of any fortifications, but an old pillar, reputed to be the coronation stone, still sits at the top of the hill. Compare this hill to the "Dragon Hills" mentioned in the Somerset and Wiltshire tour in Chapter Three.

Continue south taking the second left which crosses the T35, and then take the first left on a minor road after the T35. Proceed north through Walterstown, across the L5 through Hayes by the hostel at the Bridge of Boyne (see under *Hiking*), and then right, south, on to the L21; then left, north, on the T2 to Slane (L). Three miles to the east of Slane, on a loop road to the south of the T26 lies the Brugh na Boinne, burial place of the kings. These burials are early Bronze Age tombs, some four thousand years old. There are three burial areas: Knowth, Newgrange, and Dowth, each is about a mile away from the others. Of the three, Newgrange is the most famous and is the only one that has been completely excavated.

Newgrange in Ireland, Stonehenge in England and Carnac in Brittany are the three greatest Megalithic monuments. Newgrange seems ridiculously huge to have been just the burial place of only a few bodies; it is in the shape of a mound, with a passageway leading into the centre; a little opening above the doorway at dawn at the winter solstice directs a beam of light all the way back into the centre of the tomb where the bodies were interred. Like Stonehenge, Newgrange must have had magical or religious significance for ancient people. The other two monuments on this loop road, Knowth and Dowth, are also worth seeing, if you are allowed in, because they are in various stages of excavation and give you a true idea of the work of the archaeologist.

Go back to the T26 from Slane. A little further east along this road after the turning to the burials is a road to the left, north, that goes up to Mellifont, both to the village and to the ruins of the first Cistercian monastery in Ireland where some interesting excavations are being carried out. There is a hostel near the ruins (see under *Hiking*) and only four miles away along minor roads is Monasterboice, the ruin of an ancient monastery which probably dates from the end of the fifth century, shortly after St Patrick, the patron saint of Ireland, brought Christianity to the island. There are some high crosses, and a round tower which you can climb.

These are alternative routes; the road by Newgrange loops around back on to the T26 several miles before the town of Drogheda. You pass Oldbridge where the Battle of the Boyne was fought in 1690, in which King William III defeated James II and won the crown of England. Follow the T26 east into Drogheda (L), an energetic town that can seem too much like civilization after all that biking. A *seisiun* is held at the Boyne Valley Hotel on Wednesday nights.

Drogheda to Dublin (30 miles)

At Drogheda you can take a train to Dublin, but if you are not in a hurry you could pedal south to Dublin down the L6. If you really are a glutton for punishment, you can take an alternative bike route south via Fourknocks—an important group of Megalithic passage graves with some fine ornate rock carvings. Follow the L6 for about eight miles south (until about two miles to the north of Naul) and bear right on a minor road for Fourknocks. From there you go left, south, on a minor road to the L89 which you follow south into Dublin and the end of the bike tour.

HIKING

A WALK IN THE WICKLOWS

The Wicklows, with their chain of nine hostels spread throughout the mountains and glens, provide some of the best walking country in Ireland. The following four-day tour follows minor roads and tracks, but there is also plenty of hill climbing and walking, especially around Glenbride Hostel. The Irish One-Inch Ordnance Survey map of the Wicklows should be used for hikes here.

1. *Knockree Hostel to Tiglin Hostel (17 miles)*

From Knockree Hostel at Enniskerry go past Powerscourt on to the Old Coach Road south through Sraghmore and close by Lough Dan; head south-east through Roundwood (L), across the T61 and on to the L161 for about half a mile until you meet a minor road branching right, south. Follow this road for two miles until the intersection with the Avonmore/Ashford road where you turn left towards Ashford. The Tiglin Hostel is three miles down this road.

2. *Tiglin Hostel to Glendalough (7 miles)*

From Tiglin turn right on the road back towards Avonmore and follow it to the crossroads where you turn left, south, to approach Trooperstown Hill (1419 feet). You follow a smaller road west, up and over the hill on to the T61 which you are obliged to follow for a mile into Laragh. From Laragh, go west on the L107 to the hostel at Glendalough. The Army uses part of this area as a firing range, so at this hostel and the following hostels *check the notice board to see if there is artillery firing in the area.*

3. *Glendalough Hostel to Glenmalur Hostel (10 miles)*

Go back on to the T61, go south on it for a mile and turn right, south, on to a minor road to the Avonberg River, where you turn right, north-west, on to another minor road up the Glenmalur to the hostel. Alternatively check with the warden at the Glendalough Hostel about a path via Derrybawn Mountain, Mullacor Mountain, Ballybraid, Drumgoff and Glenmalur Hostel (about seven miles).

4. *Glenmalur Hostel to Ballinclea Hostel (8 miles)*

Follow the track over Table Mountain into the Glen of Imail (*check for artillery firing schedules*) and to the hostel at Ballinclea.

TWO MOUNTAIN WALKS IN THE SOUTH-WEST

5. *Glanmore Lake Hostel on the Healy Pass*

Set in the midst of the rugged Caha Mountains north of Bantry Bay, these walks pass through almost Alpine scenery. Carry map 24 in the Irish Ordnance Survey Half-Inch Series.

You can climb Hungry Hill (2251 feet) by walking to the end of the Glanmore Valley and making a direct ascent.

Another good walk from the hostel is the Lauragh Horseshoe, a ridge walk. There are lovely views of sea and mountains as you walk from peak to peak. Begin by climbing Cummeennahillan Mountain, continue over Tooth Mountain, Coomacloghane, and to the head of the glen. Descend via Curroghreague and back to the hostel.

It is best to check with the warden to find out the condition paths are in before setting out.

6. *Ring of Kerry Hike (7 miles)*

The east end of the Ring provides a good day's hill climbing and walking between two hostels: the Corran Tuathail Hostel and the Black Valley Hostel. You need the Irish Ordnance Survey map, in the One-Inch-Series, of the Killarney District, and check with the warden at the hostel before setting out. Anything less detailed than the one-inch map could be more confusing and dangerous in the mountains than it would be helpful. Allow plenty of daylight hours for this hike and carry a map and compass. I recommend this walk for experienced hill-walkers only.

A little distance from the Corran Tuathail Hostel is a footbridge crossing the Gaddagh River. Follow this to a trackway which traverses the glen up to the twin lakes of Gouragh and Callee. All around are huge peaks and above the path to the right, are the Hag's Teeth and the cliffs of Carrauntoohil. From the lakes cross a moor and then climb the difficult Devil's Ladder to the saddle of Carrauntoohil from which an easy grass slope leads to the summit at 3414 feet. To get to the Black Valley Hostel you do not have to go all the way to the top, but it would be a shame to get so far and not reach the summit. Go back down to the saddle at the Devil's Ladder and descend to Cummeennduf Glen via Curraghmore West, and reach the Black Valley Hostel by the track from there.

You can hire bikes at Corran Tuathail Hostel and ponies at the Black Valley Hostel.

A WALK IN CONNEMARA

7. *Ben Lettery Hostel to Killary Harbour Hostel (9 miles)*

The Twelve Bens are mountains in a circular area of about six square miles which contains some of the best scenery in

Connemara. To walk from one hostel to the other takes about four hours. You need Ordnance Survey maps in the Irish One-Inch Series numbers 93 and 84; check at the hostel before setting out to see what condition the paths are in. Go carefully and take your time as there is much scree and loose rock on this route across the Bens.

Begin this walk from the Ben Lettery Hostel by climbing Ben Lettery, then Ben Bower and continue on to Benbreen. Then walk between Benbaun and Bencollaghduff to a track leading to the Lough Inagh Road, and from there to Killary. It sounds easy on paper, but allow yourself plenty of daylight hours for the journey: not for beginners.

TWO HIKES IN DONEGAL

8. *Slieve League: Carrick Hostel to Malin Moore (12 miles)*
The village of Carrick is three miles north-west of Kilcar and is a centre for climbing Slieve League, where there is the most dramatic cliff scenery I have ever seen. At one point the cliffs drop over one thousand feet straight down into the Atlantic and there are fantastic views on every side.

Take a minor road south from Carrick for two miles to Teelin, a small village with a Gaelic college. From Teelin there is a small road up over Carrigan Head to the cliffs of Bunglass, and from here you must traverse a narrow path called One Man's Pass: on one side of this ridge is the ocean 1800 feet down and on the other is a steep precipice (the old "caught between the devil and the deep blue sea" adage is most appropriate here). But once across this pass, it is only a short distance to the top of Slieve League, 1972 feet, and you will be rewarded with enough views to have made the climb worthwhile. On a clear day they say you can see America from the summit of Slieve League.

Return to Carrick by the same route, or continue on to the village of Malin Beg to the west, and then around the shores of Malin Bay to Malin Moore (L) which is a pretty little village; there are many prehistoric tombs in the surrounding area.

Use the Irish Ordnance Survey One-Inch map number 22. Be careful of the winds, especially when crossing One Man's Pass—the wind here can pick you right off your feet if it is blowing hard off the sea. Also beware of changes in the weather. The mists can blow in very quickly so know where you are and where you are going and do not stray from the paths, especially near the cliffs. Check at Carrick Hostel before you set out about paths and weather conditions.

9. *Walks from Errigal Hostel*

The hostel is situated in the Poisoned Glen at the foot of Mount Errigal in North Donegal. This is one of the best centres in Ireland for hill walking or rock climbing. The south-west flanks of the Derryveagh Mountains to the south and the Poisoned Glen itself are rock climbing areas.

For hikers, there is Mount Errigal itself, a whitish cone of quartzite, and, at 2466 feet, Donegal's highest mountain. A direct ascent can be made to the top from Dunlewy Lake; and there is a great day's walking along the ridges north from Mount Errigal to Aghla Mor, Aghla Beag and Muckish.

Use the Irish Ordnance Survey One-Inch map number 9 and check with the hostel warden for any specially detailed walking maps he may have for sale or loan.

A WALK IN THE BOYNE VALLEY

10. *Bridge of Boyne Hostel to Mellifont Hostel (8 miles)*

The Boyne Valley is rich in history, and the two hostels provide good centres for the exploration of the tombs of Newgrange and the abbeys of Mellifont and Monasterboice (see page 136). This is a good route for beginners.

From the Bridge of Boyne Hostel walk east along the river through Beauparc and Slane. There is a tradition that on the nearby Hill of Slane, St Patrick defied paganism by lighting the Paschal Fire on the eve of Easter AD 433. In effect, St Patrick probably usurped a pagan festival that occurred at about the same time as the Christian Easter. From Slane you take the old Navan-Drogheda canal walk to the Obelisk Bridge and thence to Mellifont.

Use the Irish Ordnance Survey One-Inch map number 91, although on this walk you really have no need of a super-detailed map as you will be on flat land all the way, following the river to Slane and the canal from there to Mellifont. Check with the warden at the Boyne hostel for exact directions and current condition of the path. The walk is best done in the early part of the year: by mid-summer the tow-path to the canal is heavily overgrown.

SEVEN
The Midlands

One has no great hopes from Birmingham.
I always say there is something direful in the sound.

JANE AUSTEN: Emma

Like Jane Austen I have no great hopes for Birmingham, but the rest of the Midlands are not necessarily all "dark, satanic mills" and, contrary to popular legend, the area is not covered by smog: you will find peaceful country lanes in the Midlands just as elsewhere.

This area was the home of some interesting people: good old crusty Dr Samuel Johnson was born at Lichfield, just north-east of Birmingham; the Byron ancestral home was at Newstead Abbey, and the home of D. H. Lawrence was at Eastwood—both places are just north of Robin Hood's Nottingham. To the north-east of Nottingham, is Woolsthorpe, once the home of Sir Isaac Newton.

To the north-west of Nottingham is a national park, the Peak District, and one look at this lovely and traditional countryside will remove all preconceptions of the Midlands. The Peak District gives great variety within a small area. The southern part of the park is called the White Peak because of the rolling limestone uplands set off by wooded dales; the northern part is the Dark Peak which are gloomy and exposed moorlands. And just an hour away from this wilderness lives a population of some twenty million people.

I include a bike route in this chapter that skirts the Welsh border country. This is a connecting route from Hereford to Chester, which is also the last town of the "exit" tour from Wales. However, the main bike route of the Midlands is in the Peak District, about forty miles to the east of Chester. This is a fairly easy route including lovely old villages with ancient customs, famous mansions and caves.

In the south of the Peak District there is a hike route on the

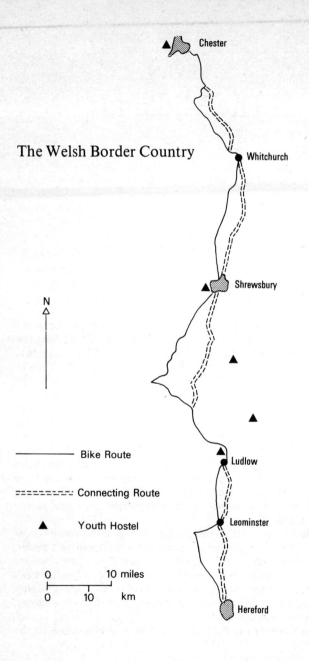

The Welsh Border Country

Chester

Whitchurch

Shrewsbury

Ludlow

Leominster

Hereford

N

———— Bike Route

========= Connecting Route

▲ Youth Hostel

0   10 miles

0   10   km

Tissington and High Peak disused railway line which coincides well with the biking route in the same area. There is also, in the, north of the park, some fifteen miles of the long distance route called the Pennine Way. However, as most of this long and difficult trail is in the North of England, the description of the route is given in Chapter Eight.

The bike routes in the Midlands are covered by maps 10, 11 and 13 in the Ordnance Survey Quarter-Inch Series, and by maps 13, 18, 23, 24, 28 and 29 in the Bartholomew 1:100,000 Series.

BIKING

THE WELSH BORDER COUNTRY
(100 miles)

This tour goes through Herefordshire, Salop (the abbreviation for Shropshire), and into Cheshire. Along the length of this route you will see typical traditional English scenery: from the black-and-white half-timbered houses of Shropshire to the medieval walled city of Chester.

Hereford to Chester (100 miles)

From the cathedral city of Hereford it is about twenty-three miles to Ludlow across the meadows of Hereford and into Salop. Take the A4110 north out of Hereford to the intersection with the A4112 where you turn right, north-east into Leominster, a medieval town that acquired its wealth through the wool trade; walk along the narrow streets with their overhanging half-timbered, Elizabethan buildings. From Leominster take a minor road north towards Orleton. By-pass Orleton by avoiding any turns off the minor road till it intersects with A49 about two miles south of Ludlow. Follow the A49 into Ludlow (HL), a small town with black and white half-timbered buildings surrounding a castle and cathedral. This was one of the border outposts between England and Wales in the days of the border chieftains: see the elegant carving of the Feathers, a Tudor inn.

From Ludlow it is thirty-five miles via backroads to Shrewsbury (HC). Take the A49 north for about eight miles to the A189 turning to the left, north-west, which you take to Lydham. From

Lydham take a minor road north-east all the way into Shrewsbury. Shrewsbury is one of the best preserved of medieval towns in England; it was originally built by the Romans, later the Normans moved in which accounts for the castle. There are multitudes of amazing street names: see especially Butcher Row, Wyle Cap, Fish Street, Grope Lane and Dogpole, as these streets contain some of the best black and white half-timbered buildings.

It is forty-two miles to Chester from Shrewsbury going via Whitchurch. You can venture into Wales from Shrewsbury and travel to Betws-y-Coed and from there follow the Welsh bike route out to Chester (see Chapter Five).

Otherwise, take the A528 north out of Shrewsbury, past Hadnall where you take minor road to the right, north, for Wem. Continue through Wem and Tilstock into Whitchurch; from here take the A41 a couple of miles north till you reach a minor road branching off to the left, north-west. This takes you through Malpas, Tilson, across the A534 and back on to the A41 going north for a further seven miles into Chester (HLC, see Chapter Five).

THE PEAK DISTRICT
(100 miles)

Buxton to Bakewell (50 miles)
This tour begins in the south of the Peak District. Buxton can be reached by train from Chester. Buxton (HLC) is the centre of the Peak District, a town of about twenty thousand people; it was originally a spa, supposed at one time to rival Bath. Mary Queen of Scots was treated for rheumatism here. There is a *well-dressing* ceremony at Buxton in the summer, well-dressing being a pagan ceremony (taken over by the church) during which the wells are decorated to give thanks for a plentiful water supply. This custom is peculiar to Derbyshire.

From Buxton go south-east on the A515 for five miles, then bear right on to the B5053 going south through Longnor and Warslow; continue south-west on the B5053 to meet the A523 where you turn left, south-east for Ashbourne (C). Ashbourne is the southern gateway to the Peak District National Park. It is a small market town, quiet and pleasant: see the almshouses in the main street, also the church and spire; Johnson and Boswell stayed at the Green Man Hotel. (See under *Hiking.*)

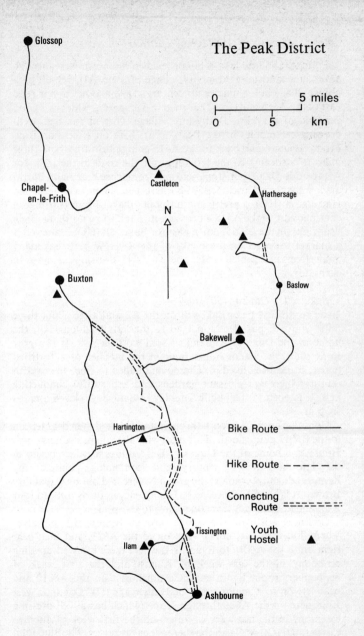

The Peak District

Glossop

Chapel-en-le-Frith

Castleton

Hathersage

N

Buxton

Baslow

Bakewell

Hartington

Bike Route ——————

Hike Route – – – – –

Connecting Route

Youth Hostel ▲

Tissington

Ilam

Ashbourne

0   5 miles

0   5 km

From Ashbourne take a minor road to the north-west through Mappleton and into the pretty village of Ilam (H), rebuilt as a model village in the nineteenth century. Take another minor road east to the A515 and cross that road to Tissington, which is a good example of a typical Derbyshire village. One of the best well-dressing ceremonies in the Peak occurs here on Ascension Day. From Tissington go back to the A515 going north for about three miles to a turning to the left (opposite the road to the right for Alsop-en-le-Dale) to Alstonefield and from there bear right, north, on a minor road to the B5054 where you again bear right for Hartington (HC), a pretty and unspoilt village. From Hartington continue east to the A515 where you turn left to go north and then bear right on the B5055, north-east for Bakewell (HC). Bakewell is a market town set on the banks of the River Wye. It has many quiet streets and gabled roofs. There is a well-dressing ceremony in early July.

Bakewell to Glossop (50 miles)

Head south-east from Bakewell on the A6 and after about three miles you will pass Haddon Hall to the left. Haddon Hall, the home of the Duke of Rutland, is well worth a visit. It is a grey stone medieval manor house built in the manner of a fortified house; it has been lived in, altered and added to since the twelfth century; there are pleasant gardens and a beautiful banqueting hall. It is open to the public Tuesday to Saturday, eleven a.m. to six p.m.

Continue on the A6 south through Rowsley and then bear left on to the B6012 going north. This road will take you past Chatsworth House, the home of the Dukes of Devonshire, a palace begun in the late seventeenth century and containing paintings by Rembrandt and Reynolds; the grounds were laid out by Capability Brown. It is open Wednesday to Friday, eleven-thirty a.m. to four p.m. and at weekends from one-thirty to five p.m.

Continue north on the B6012 through Baslow (L) to Calver where you turn left, north-west, on to the A623, and then bear right on to the A6010 to Eyam (H), where there is a well-dressing ceremony in the last week of August and the first week of September. From Eyam continue north-east on the A6010 and bear left on to a minor road for Hathersage (H). Continue west from here on the A625 through Hope (which has a well-dressing ceremony in the last week of June and the first week of July) to Castleton (HC). At Castleton there are caves galore. The Blue John

Caverns and Mine are well worth a visit; *blue john* is a translucent fluorspar which has red, blue, yellow and purple veins.

From Castleton continue west on the A625 for Chapel-en-le-Frith (L), a little market town on the edge of what used to be the Forest of the Peak. There are some nice old inns and stocks in the square. Continue north on the A624 through Hayfield to Glossop (L), a busy industrial town which ends the tour of the Peaks. This town is set on the moors and is a favourite centre for rambles. There are train connections at Glossop.

HIKING

TISSINGTON and HIGH PEAK TRAILS
(16 miles)

There are two trails in the south of the Peak District Park which follow old railway tracks, so they are suitable for pony trekking and biking as well as hiking. These two trails meet at the point where the Tissington Trail ends. So I combine the two routes into one path to make a hike of some sixteen miles from Ashbourne in the south, to Hurdlow in the north.

This path is suitable for beginners and is so easy to follow that no description is needed. The path goes near or through the villages of Thorpe, Tissington, Alsop-en-le-Dale and Hartington. Use the Ordnance Survey Tourist Map of the Peak District.

EIGHT
The North of England

Bright and fierce and fickle is the South,
And dark and true and tender is the North.

ALFRED, LORD TENNYSON: The Princess

The North Country is a vast touring region, and the eastern portion of it, especially around the Yorkshire Moors and the city of York is one of my all-time favourites for touring. The whole region has the richest variety of scenery to be found anywhere in the British Isles. There is wild moorland, gentle dales, mountain lakeland and seacoast. What more could you want? There are four national parks and the Yorkshire Dales and North Yorkshire Moors are largely undiscovered; in fact, except in the Lake District which is world famous and also world-crowded, you can avoid high season crowds and deny yourself none of the traditional sights of the North of England.

It is assumed that the North of England will be a gateway to Scotland, so I have developed the flow of the routes to take you from the Midlands through the North-West of England and into the Lowlands of Scotland; and the route down through the North-East follows the "exit" route from Scotland.

There are five bike routes, taking you through all sorts of scenery and through all the national parks; there are two long distance paths and two shorter routes.

The bike routes in the North of England are covered by maps 7, 8, 9, 10 and 11 in the Ordnance Survey Quarter-Inch Series, and by maps 32, 33, 34, 35, 36, 39 and 42 in the Bartholomew 1:100,000 Series.

BIKING

BRONTË COUNTRY and THE YORKSHIRE DALES
(85 miles)

This is a connecting route from the Midlands to the North Country. It takes you through the rugged moorland country where the four Brontë children grew up, and which shaped much of their writing. Further north the route goes through pleasant little villages into the rolling dales of Yorkshire. The moors provide some rough riding, but overall the route is not a severe test.

Hebden Bridge to Kettlewell (45 miles)

Hebden Bridge (CL) is about twenty-five miles north of Glossop where the bike route for the Midlands ends and there are rail connections. The town is a good centre for the surrounding hills, moors and wooded valleys. There are attractive little villages such as Heptonstall and Cragy Head in the vicinity.

From Hebden Bridge take the A6033 north to Haworth (L) and into the heart of Brontë country. The Brontës came here in 1820 when Patrick Brontë brought his wife and family of six children to live at Haworth parsonage. The mother and two eldest children died during the first five years of residence leaving Patrick Brontë with the remaining children, Charlotte, Emily, Branwell and Anne. The four children grew up in semi-isolation in the midst of these rugged Pennine Moors, and once you see the setting of their lives you will immediately understand the musings that went into the writing of their novels. Even as children, these four would invent stories and people to wile away the long winter days.

The parsonage at Haworth is now a museum (open eleven a.m. to six p.m. every day except Sunday). The rooms are arranged as they were when Emily, Anne, and Charlotte lived and wrote there. Branwell, the failure of the family, died, an alcoholic and opium addict in 1848, and Emily and Anne died of consumption in the following year. Charlotte lived on until 1855, dying when she was thirty-nine, just one year after her marriage. About four miles from Haworth, at Far Withens, is the site of Emily's *Wuthering Heights,* and the nearby ruins of Wycollen Hall were probably the setting for Ferndean Hall in Charlotte's classic, *Jane Eyre.* Lowood School from the same novel is Cowan Bridge.

From Haworth continue north on the A6033 through Keighley,

Brontë Country and the Yorkshire Dales

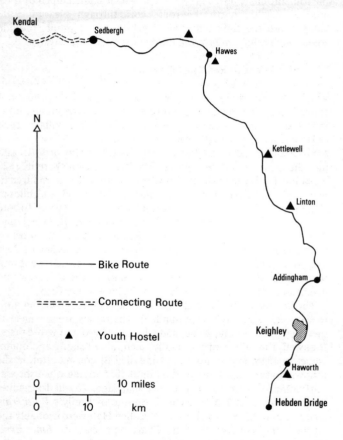

bear left on the A650, and then right on the 6034 for Addingham. From Addingham, take the B6160 north across the A59, past Bolton Abbey (L) to Bardon Tower where you turn right on to a minor road and then left so that you are travelling north parallel to the B6160. Continue through the little village of Appletreewick which is packed with sixteenth-century gabled cottages and a population of two hundred. Keep north on the minor road past Nearby Burnsall (on the B6160) to Hebden (L), Grassington (H, two miles away on the B6160; C), and continue to Cornistone where you bear left, west, for half a mile back to the B6160 where you turn right, north, into Kettlewell (H).

You are now in the Yorkshire Dales where some of the valleys are easy and rolling and others are harsh-cut ravines. The Dales are a National Park; the area is also referred to as the West Riding. The county of Yorkshire is divided into three *Ridings* from the Scandinavian *Thrydding* meaning one-third, for much of the North was settled by Norsemen at the time of the Viking raids.

Kettlewell to Sedbergh (40 miles)
From Kettlewell take the B6160 north to Buckden through the beautiful Wharfdale. At Buckden take a minor road to the left, north-west, through Hubberholme and along the Langstrothdale to the village of Deepdale. Continue north on the same minor road all the way to Hawes (HCL). (See under *Hiking*: the Pennine Way.) From Hawes take the B6255 south-west for about seven miles until a right turn on to a minor road past the hostel at Dentdale. Continue west through Lea Yeat along the Dentdale to Dent (L); then take a minor road north-west through Millthrop to Sedbergh (CL) and the end of the tour.

THE LAKE DISTRICT
(120 miles)

It can be hard going sometimes in Lakeland, with the mountainous country and many tourists and holiday-makers. From the previous tour of the Dales, it is a short ten miles by bike from Sedbergh on the A684, west, to the starting point of this tour at Kendal. Kendal is the gateway to the Lake District National Park, which is one of the most popular parks in England, and, at 886 square miles, one of the largest. The Lakeland countryside is beautiful, and marvellous for walking. There are literary associations with the

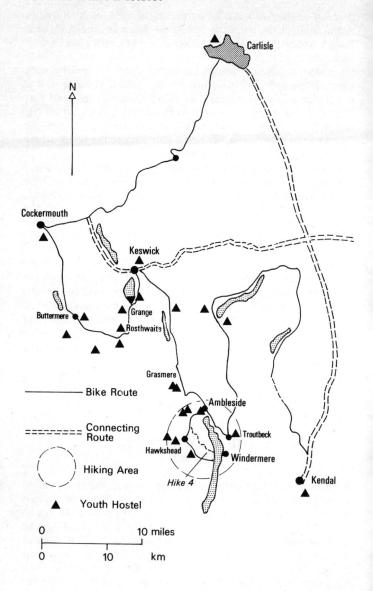

The Lake District

N

Carlisle

Cockermouth

Keswick

Buttermere

Grange

Rosthwaite

Grasmere

Ambleside

Troutbeck

Hawkshead

Windermere

Hike 4

Kendal

——— Bike Route

‑ ‑ ‑ ‑ Connecting
Route

◯ Hiking Area

▲ Youth Hostel

0   10 miles

0   10   km

Romantic Poets: William Wordsworth, Samuel Taylor Coleridge, Percy Bysshe Shelley and John Keats, who all praised the scenery of the lakes in one poem or another.

Kendal to Troutbeck Bridge (50 miles)

From the market town of Kendal (HL) proceed north on a minor road to Burnside where you turn right, north-east, on to another minor road to Garnett Bridge. From here go north on a road to Sadgill, where the road ends, the paved one at least, but there is a mountain track of about four miles to the resumption of the road near Hawes Water. There are stretches along this track where you will have to wheel your bike. Once back on the road, continue north-east through Bampton (L) and Askham. At Askham you turn left on to a minor road going west for Pooley Bridge (LC). Go through that town and take the right fork for the A592. Turn left, south-west, on the A592 along the lake of Ullswater into Patterdale (H). Continue south on the A592 over Kirkstone Pass to Troutbeck, where you turn right off the A592 and go through the middle of the village set in this fine valley. Continue south on the minor road past the hostel to Troutbeck Bridge.

Troutbeck Bridge to Cockermouth (40 miles)

Take the A591 north-west to Ambleside (HLC) on the head of Britain's largest lake—Windermere (see under *Hiking*). Ambleside is a quiet little village, much frequented in the last century by Wordsworth, Coleridge, and the writer, John Ruskin. Continue north on the A591 to Grasmere (L) on the lake of the same name. This is another tiny village which can be jam-packed with tourists in the summer: see Dove Cottage, formerly the home of Wordsworth and now a museum devoted to that poet. He is buried in Grasmere Churchyard.

Take the A591 north from Grasmere to the tip of Thirlmere lake where you turn left on to a minor road which will take you along the west side of the lake. This road forks at the northern end of the lake and you bear left to rejoin the A591 to Keswick (HLC), which is a touring centre for the lakes and usually quite busy; it is a pretty little town with twisting streets. The poet Coleridge lived at Greta Hall nearby.

From Keswick proceed south on the B5289 through Grange (H) and Rosthwaite (HL) a dabble of houses in the peaks. The road veers to the right here, to the west, to climb over the steep Honister Pass (H); then along Lake Buttermere and into the village of Buttermere (HL), another tiny group of houses amidst the peaks and lakes: a good centre for the Cumbrian Mountains. From Buttermere continue north on the B5289 past the village of High Lorton and on into Cockermouth (CLH). This is a larger market town, the birthplace of William Wordsworth, also of Fletcher Christian, who led the mutiny on the *Bounty*.

Cockermouth to Carlisle (30 miles)

Take the A66 east out of Cockermouth for five miles to where the B5291 turns off to the left. Follow the B5291 through Kilnhill and bear right on a minor road, east, for Bassenthwaite (LC). Continue through that village, north, on the same minor road until it joins the B5299, right, to Caldbeck. Continue north on a minor road from Caldbeck turning sharply right after a few miles on to another minor road, through Rosley Welton, Darlston and into Carlisle (HLC). This is a large town near the western end of the Emperor Hadrian's well-known wall fortification (see under *Hiking*). From this city there is easy access to the Lowlands of Scotland (see Chapter Nine) or there are rail connections from here to the eastern region of the North Country for the next tour in this chapter.

NORTHUMBERLAND
(140 miles)

This is mainly a connecting route between the Scottish Lowlands and the more southerly routes, though you do pass through some lovely scenery.

Berwick upon Tweed to Alnwick (40 miles)

From Berwick (LC), a busy market town encircled by ancient walls, proceed south on the A1 for eleven miles until you reach the Beal turning to the left. From Beal (C), at low tide, you can reach Holy Island, by a causeway. This island was a cradle of Christianity in those dark years after the collapse of the Roman Empire (See Chapters Three and Six). There is a little village on the island, the remains of a monastery, and the ruins of an eleventh-century Benedictine priory. Lindisfarne Mead, a strong honey wine once drunk by the monks, is still brewed on the island.

Return to Beal and go back on to the A1 turning left, to go south, for about five miles to Belford (C) where you again bear left, east, to Bamburgh (LC). Continue along the coast to

Seahouses (L) and Beadnell (C). Turn inland at Beadnell on a minor road south-west for two miles and then left again on a minor road south through Embleton, and Longhoughton where you turn right into Alnwick (L). This is the county town of Northumberland and has an excellent castle dating from the twelfth century, which is open to the public in the afternoons.

Alnwick to Chollerford (38 miles)

Take the B6341 out of Alnwick going south-west to Rothbury (LC) in the Dale of Coquet. Continue on minor roads in a general south-west direction through Thropton, Hepple, and across part of the Northumberland National Park through Elsdon (L) to Otterburn (L). In 1388 Otterburn was the scene of the moonlit battle between the Scots and the English which was immortalized in Sir Walter Scott's ballad *Chevy Chase*. See the Otterburn Tweed factory while you are here.

Take a minor road south-west from Otterburn for two miles to connect with the A68 where you turn left to go south through Ridsdale to the junction with the A6079 where you turn right for Chollerford, a good centre from which to explore Hadrian's Wall (see under *Hiking*).

Chollerford to Darlington (60 miles)

Go south from Chollerford on the A6079 through Acomb (H) to Hexham (LC), a market town on the River Tyne. The Abbey church and ruins at Hexham date from 673. After Hexham, stay on minor roads south through Slaley to the village of Blanchland (L), a fine site in the valley of the Derwent. While you are there have a pint at the Lord Crewe Arms; the inn is haunted by a mysterious spectre—the adventurous may want to spend a night there! There are more hills after Blanchland and the going gets tougher. Stay on a minor road east to Edmundbyers (H), then go south across the A689 through Stanhope (C) to Eggleston, then across the River Tees to Romaldkirk in Teesdale. Continue south-east along the River Tees to Barnard Castle (H) a little market town which has connections with Charles Dickens; there is also a twelfth-century castle on the cliff overlooking the River Tees. From Barnard Castle go north-east on the A67 and stay on this road for about seventeen miles to Darlington (L), a large town steeped in railway history; the town is full of engineering shops which British Rail closed down in 1966. Darlington is the end of this route and puts you in a good position to start the next tour

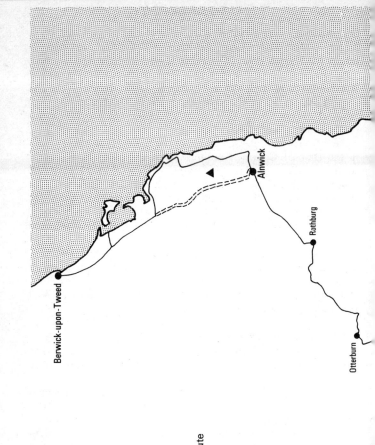

Northumberland

———— Bike Route

======== Connecting Route

– – – – Hike Route

▲ Youth Hostel

□ Ruins

Berwick-upon-Tweed

Alnwick

Rothbury

Otterburn

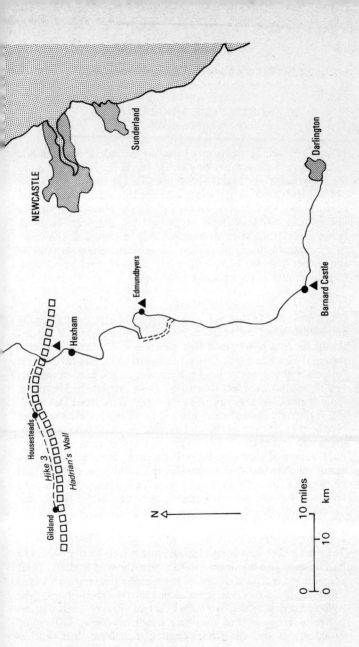

across the North York Moors to the city of York.

NORTH YORK MOORS to YORK
(85 miles)

If you are joining this route from the preceding Northumbria route, you can pedal the twenty-five miles via the A67, right on to the A19, then left on to the A1044, going east all the way.

The first fifty miles of the tour take you through a major section of the North York Moors National Park. The northern moors are not quite so wild as those in Devon, but they can be bleak nonetheless. If the skies are blue you may be rewarded with views of the heather all purple against the horizon. The going can be rough, but the tours keep to the river valleys as much as possible. (See under *Hiking* for walks on the Moor.)

Stokesley to Helmsley (50 miles)

From Stokesley (L) set out on a minor road east through Easby and Kildale and Commondale. Just past Commondale turn right, south, on to a minor road that passes near Castleton and goes through Westerdale (H). Stay on this road south and take a right fork after about three miles for Farndale. At the head of the dale you should take the left fork to go along the dale to Hutton-le-Hole. This route takes you along the banks of the River Dove and, if it is the right time of year, you will be all but knocked off your bike by the yellow of all the wild daffodils—sorry, but it is against the law to pick them. You will come out of Farndale at the story-book village of Hutton-le-Hole. From here you travel south on a minor road through Kirkbymoorside (L), another lovely moorland village, and on to the A170 going west for Helmsley (HL), a small market town with a twelfth century castle (see under *Hiking*: the Cleveland Way).

Helmsley to York (35 miles)

Take the B1257 west from Helmsley and turn left after two and a half miles on to a minor road to Rievaulx Abbey in Ryedale. There you will see the ruins of one of the greatest Cistercian abbeys in England. The abbey was founded in 1131 by French monks who followed their Norman overlords over from France. In its day this powerful abbey housed over five hundred people. The monks raised money to build from donations and from their skills as sheep farmers: at its height, the abbey had at least twelve thousand sheep on the moors. However, the great wealth of this monastery and others like it (they owned one-third of England by the sixteenth century) in addition to their obedience to Rome, was their undoing. Henry VIII had little trust in or love for religious institutions which rivalled the power of the state. In 1536, in the Act of Dissolution, he dissolved all monastic foundations. Rievaulx, like so many others, was dissolved, abandoned and left to decay, which it has done most gracefully.

From Rievaulx Abbey follow minor roads west and south through Old Byland, passing nearby Cold Kirby, then on to the A170 (a left turn) for half a mile to another minor road where you turn right, south, through Kilburn, to Coxwold (L), a lovely little village of two hundred people. Shandy Hall, not far from the village, is an ordinary brick house, the home of Laurence Sterne and where he wrote part of *Tristram Shandy* in 1769. Continue south on minor roads past Newburgh Priory, through Oulston and Huby to meet the B1363 at Sutton-on-the-Forest. Follow the B1363 south into the city of York (HLC, five miles south).

York is a small but really lovely city with old winding streets, called the Shambles, where the houses lean over on both sides. Try Ye Olde Starre Inne in Stonegate for a delicious pub lunch in a fine old oak-beamed pub. York looks amazingly medieval with high grey stone walls still encircling it, and with the cathedral, York Minster, dwarfing all the surrounding buildings: see the excellent stained glass in the cathedral, especially the east window, where 117 square yards of glass panels tell the story of the Bible from the Creation to the Apocalypse. The York Mystery Plays, a fourteenth century cycle of miracle plays taken from the Bible, are performed every third year. There is also a very good repertory theatre—one of the best in England; and do not miss the Castle Museum. All in all, there are nowhere near enough superlatives to describe the city of York.

Routes around York

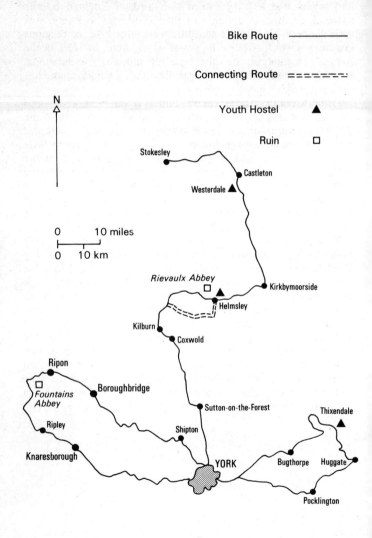

Bike Route ───────

Connecting Route ========

Youth Hostel ▲

Ruin □

N

0 ⊢—— 10 miles
0 ⊢—— 10 km

Stokesley

Castleton

Westerdale ▲

Rievaulx Abbey □

▲ Helmsley

Kirkbymoorside

Kilburn

Coxwold

Ripon

Fountains
Abbey □

Boroughbridge

Ripley

Sutton-on-the-Forest

Knaresborough

Shipton

Thixendale ▲

YORK

Bugthorpe

Huggate

Pocklington

TWO ROUTES AROUND YORK
(55 miles and 50 miles)

If you like York, as I think you will, you may want to stay there for a few days and use it as a centre for tours in the surrounding area. Here are two circular routes from York.

York to Fountains Abbey and back (55 miles)

Leave York on the A19 going north to Shipton. Here you turn left on to a minor road through Newton-on-Ouse. Continue north-west for another seven miles till you bear right at a turning for Boroughbridge (L). Continue through Boroughbridge and across the A1 on the same minor road into Ripon (L), a small cathedral city which still keeps up the medieval curfew custom of blowing a horn in the square at nine p.m. Take the B6265 west out of Ripon for two miles and turn left on to a minor road for Fountains Abbey. This abbey, like Rievaulx farther to the north was built by the Cistercians and fell into decay after Henry VIII's Act of Dissolution (see page 161). It is considered to be one of the most outstanding monastic ruins in Western Europe.

From here go south on minor roads to Ripley, then take the B6165 south-east to Knaresborough (L) with its river gorge and caves. Take the B6164 south from Knaresborough and bear left after four miles on to a minor road which crosses the A1 and leads you through Cowthorpe and Tockwith to Long Marston and the B1224. Follow the B1224 east back into York.

York to the Wolds and back (50 miles)

The Wolds here are a forty mile long chalk hump, from four hundred to eight hundred feet high. Nearby is some of the most fertile land in England and there are some lovely villages set in pastoral countryside.

Take the A166 north-east out of York through Stamford Bridge (C). Turn off to the left on a minor road three miles past Stamford Bridge for Bugthorpe, and continue on this minor road east through Kirby Underdale. Take a hard left, north, about one and a half miles beyond Kirby to skirt the Wold. This minor road goes north and you must turn hard right to the south for Aldro then continue south from there on to Thixendale (H), a pleasant village in the Wolds. Continue south from Thixendale across the A166 to Huggate and from there south-west on a minor road for Millington, through Pocklington (L) and on to the B1246 west through Barmby Moor; just west of here you bear right on to the A1079 which takes you back west into York.

HIKING

There are plenty of hikes in the North Country. Two long distance paths, both fairly difficult give many miles of challenging walking and climbing; and two shorter walks—one along Hadrian's Wall and another in the Lake District—provide easier and shorter routes. Portions of the long distance routes could provide an enjoyable day's walk.

THE PENNINE WAY
(250 miles)

This is the longest and the most rugged of any of the long distance paths in Britain. It stretches from the Peak District in the south to the Cheviot Hills on the Scottish Border. The path runs along the Pennine Range, sometimes called the backbone of England. It was the first long-distance path to be opened and combines old Roman roads, miners' and shepherds' tracks and old footpaths into one long public right of way. Some of the roughest hiking in England is to be found on the Pennine Way. It is definitely not for beginners (though there are some easy stretches), so do not attempt it unless you have experience of plotting a course with map and compass. The way is marked with signposts in oak displaying the acorn symbol. Display boards containing large-scale maps are mounted at intervals along the way. Maps in the Ordnance Survey 150,000 Series are 74, 80, 86, 91, 92, 98, 103, 109, 110. A useful guidebook is *Walking the Pennine Way* by Alan P. Binns, published by Gerrard Publications.

Along most of the length of the Pennine Way there are lodgings within one or two miles of the path. But at the northern end there is a twenty-seven mile stretch between Byrness and Kirk Yetholm that you must do in one day unless you have camping equipment. There are many hostels along the path.

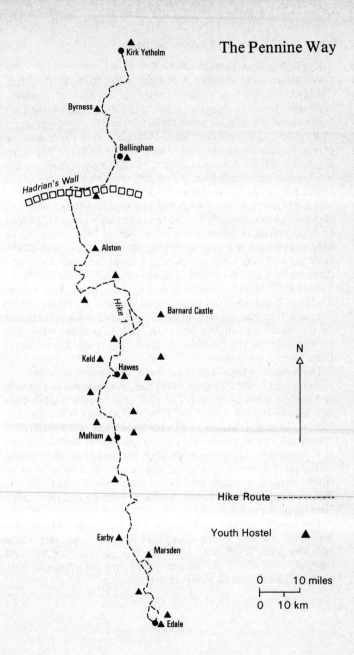

The Pennine Way

Kirk Yetholm

Byrness

Bellingham

Hadrian's Wall

Alston

Hike 1

Barnard Castle

Keld
Hawes

Malham

N

Hike Route ----------

Youth Hostel ▲

Earby
Marsden

0   10 miles
0   10 km

Edale

1. *Edale to Kirk Yetholm (250 miles)*

I will describe the Pennine Way from south to north though it would obviously be just as easy to negotiate it from north to south.

Starting from the village of Edale in the Peak District, the path heads north over Kinder Scout (2088 feet) and into the wilderness of Bleaklow (2061 feet) and Black Hill (1908 feet). From here the path continues north through White Moss and Black Moss, by Standedge and Blackstone Edge to the Calder Valley, then into the bleak moorland of the Brontë Country, after which it crosses the lowlands of Craven into the green fields and limestone walls that encircle Malham in the Yorkshire Dales National Park. Next, the path crosses Fountains Fell (2191 feet) and Pen-y-ghent (2273 feet) as it progresses to Ribblesdale. From here a pack horse trail is followed by Cam Fell to green Wensleydale. Then the path climbs again up and over Great Shunner Fell (2340 feet) and down into the peaceful Upper Swaledale, and up again like a roller-coaster to Tan Hill (1732 feet), where you can find the highest inn in England. From here the path crosses the gap of Stainmore to Teesdale, then goes upstream past the waterfall at High Force and up the waters of Caldron Snout to High Cup Nick, where the western ridge of the Pennines drops sharply to the Eden Valley. From here the path winds into Dufton.

The summit of Cross Fell (2930 feet) is climbed next—this is the highest point in the Pennines—then the path descends to Carrigill and the old town of Alston. The path goes into South Tynedale and follows the old Roman road up to Hadrian's Wall, which it follows through its best section by the Nine Nicks of Thirlwall over Winshields and the heights above Crag Lough near the Roman fort at Housesteads. After Hadrian's Wall, the path crosses the moors and some Forestry Commission plantations as it progresses to North Tyne and Redesdale. From Redesdale it climbs to the Roman camps at Chew Green and follows the Roman road called Dere Street for a mile or so.

The last bit of the pathway follows the Border Fence over Beefstand Hill and Windy Gyle (2034 feet); then Auchope Cairn and The Schil (1985 feet) after which it joins a footpath and descends by the fine Halterburn Valley into the village of Kirk Yetholm and the end of a long, rigorous journey.

THE CLEVELAND WAY
(100 miles)

The Cleveland Way is a long distance path that runs around the borders of the North York Moors National Park, through impressive moorland scenery, and along some exhilarating cliffs on the seacoast. Some of the path, especially that portion on the moor, can be difficult, so, as with any moorland walk, you should be careful and know what you are doing.

Ordnance Survey maps in the 1:50,000 Series, numbers 93, 94, 99, 100, and 101 are needed for this walk. The way is marked along its entire length: where it leaves or joins roads there are signposts with the words *Moor Path* or *Coast Path*; away from the roads there is the acorn symbol at places where the hiker might take the wrong route. There is an official guidebook: *The Cleveland Way,* by Alan Falconer, with Ordnance Survey maps and pictures; also a rival publication published by the Dalesman Publishing Company: *The Cleveland Way,* by Bill Cowley.

There is plenty of accommodation along the coast; on the moors you may have to descend from the hills to find lodgings, so it is best to carry camping equipment for that stretch at least. There are several hostels along the route.

2. *Helmsley to Filey (100 miles)*

From the fine old market town of Helmsley (HL), the path goes west past Helmsley Castle to Whinny Bank and by the ruins of Rievaulx Abbey (see page 160) to Sutton Bank, where a short detour can be made to Roulston Scar to see some splendid views over the Plain of York to the south. The path proceeds north along Whitestone Cliff, along the edge of the Hambleton Hills and Black Hambleton to the village of Osmotherly (L). Then the path climbs Swinestye Hill, past My Lady's Chapel and by Mount Grace Priory to Arncliffe, and from there down to Scugdale Beck. The path climbs to cross the rugged country of Whorlton, Carlton and Cringle Moors, past Ingleby Moor, north across Battersby Moor and down to the village of Kildale. The path climbs from Kildale up to Easby Moor, where there is a monument to Captain Cook, and then north across Great Ayton Moor, north-east across Gisborough Moor; and then the path begins to slowly descend to the coast leaving the moors for good. The first town on the coast is Saltburn (HL).

On part of the eastern moorland and for some way south of

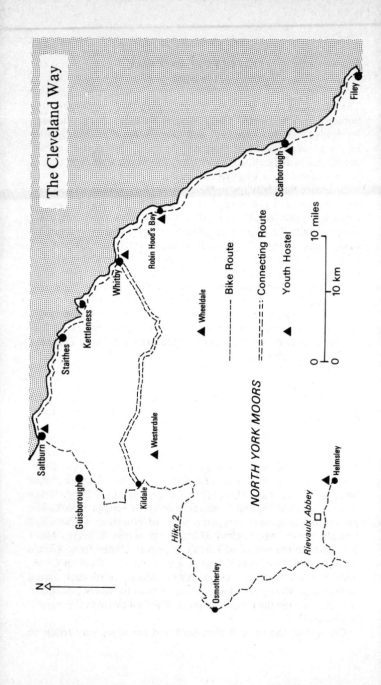

The Cleveland Way

Saltburn the path is not in the National Park. After Saltburn the path goes south along the coast and re-enters the National Park east of Skinningrove. It climbs over Boulby Hill, passes along the coastline through Staithes and Runswick Bay and over Kettleness to Whitby (LCH), one of the nicer coastal towns of Yorkshire. This is the town where the explorer Captain Cook began his sailing apprenticeship by working on the coal ships. To the south, you pass the ruins of Whitby Abbey: built in the seventh century, destroyed in the eleventh century by the Vikings, refounded and rebuilt in the same century, then dissolved and abandoned in the sixteenth century. What remains to be seen today is the work of the twelfth and thirteenth centuries.

Follow the cliff walk south from Whitby (caution is needed near the edge of the cliffs as there has been much erosion) to Robin Hood's Bay (LHC), a lovely little fishing village with steep streets tumbling down into the ocean. From Robin Hood's Bay the path continues along the cliffs to Ravenscar, south behind the cliff edge to Hayburn Wyke and then along the coast by Cloughton Wyke to the big and busy resort of Scarborough (LCH). This town was built as a spa when medicinal springs were discovered on the site in the seventeenth century. Follow the cliff top south past Cayton Sands to the boundary line of the North and East Ridings just to the north of Filey.

HADRIAN'S WALL and THE LAKE DISTRICT

It was after the Roman Emperor Hadrian's visit to Britain in AD 122 that he ordered what is now known as the Roman Wall or Hadrian's Wall to be erected as a frontier barrier. This wall stretched from Wallsend on the Tyne in the east to Bowness on the Solway in the west cutting right across the north of England. Forts, milecastles and signalling towers were built along the whole length of the wall, and garrisons were built nearby, so that the wall presented a continuous fortified line. It was originally built partly of turf, but was later reconstructed in stone. In addition to the parapets, forts and turrets, there were ditches some twenty feet wide on both sides of the wall. A garrison army of five and a half thousand cavalry and thirteen thousand infantry kept vigil against attack from the barbaric north, and, in more peaceful times, acted like a customs post, regulating trade between north and south.

Some of the best preserved sections of the wall (much of the stone of the wall was used in constructing the Military Road which runs parallel to it) as well as some of the best preserved forts, are along the sixteen mile track that the following hiking route covers. An essential map for this route is the Ordnance Survey two-inches to one mile map called, rightly enough, *Hadrian's Wall.* Be sure to wear heavy boots for this hike, as parts of it traverse rugged and hilly ground.

3. *Chollerford to Gilsland (16 miles)*

The walk begins just one mile west of Chollerford. Follow the B6318, or the Military Road, east. To the south of this road you will find Cilurnum, or Chesters, a large Roman fort from the second century; it covers about five acres and the ruins include barracks, stables and baths for the soldiers. North of the B6318 at this point the Wall begins and you can now leave the road and begin following the course of the Wall eastwards. The Wall is your waymarked path.

Brocolita, another Roman fort south of the Military Road will come into view after about three miles; four miles further on, you will come to Vercovicium, or Housesteads, again on the south side of the wall. This is one of the best examples of a Roman fort; it covers five acres and could accommodate one thousand infantry. Remains of walls, turrets and granaries can still be seen. Three miles from here and just south of the Military Road is the Once Brewed Hostel and an inn on the road nearby. Continuing east along the Wall you will come to Cawfields, one of the best examples of a milecastle. Milecastles were set up at intervals of 1620 yards (one Roman mile); they were defensive and communications posts, with two signal towers placed at equal intervals between each milecastle and the next. Not far to the east of Cawfields is Aesica or Great Chesters, another fort on the line of the Wall. Another four miles and you come into Gilsland and the end of the route.

4. *A Walk in the Lake District: Bowness on Windermere to Hawkshead (6 miles)*

The Lake District has many miles of footpaths, providing both long and short walks all over lakeland England. This area is a National Park and the park service publishes leaflets on many of these walks; describing exactly how to find your way on the paths. For example, there is an excellent eight mile walk from Keswick around its neighbouring lake, Derwent Water. At points the path does leave the lake's edge so that the pamphlet, available at the Keswick Information Centre, or an Ordnance Survey One Inch Tourist Map of the Lake District is invaluable.

The walk I include here is waymarked with white paint splashes on rocks, walls and trees and posts along the route, thus requiring little description on my part.

From Bowness, which is a Victorian resort on Lake Windermere, you take the ferry across the lake and follow the white markings from the ferry landing over Claife Heights and into Hawkshead (HL), the village where William Wordsworth attended grammar school. In summer there is a bus service that takes you back from Hawkshead to the ferry terminal. There is a nice piece of folklore concerning the path over Claife Heights. The legend says that an apparition, the "Crier of Claife", calls plaintively for a ferry boat on stormy nights from high above the lake; many of the locals still avoid tackling these heights at night. In places the ground can be wet and marshy, so you need stout boots. The going is fairly easy as you never go above the eight hundred foot level, and there are excellent views all the way.

OTHER HIKES IN THE NORTH OF ENGLAND

In the North York Moors National Park, there is the Lyke Wake Walk, a forty mile hike across the moors from Scarth Wood Moor near Osmotherly in the West to Wyke Point at Ravenscar on the east coast. Details of this hike are available from Mr W. Cowley, Potto Hill, Swainby, Northallerton, North Yorkshire; or check at park offices and bookshops in the area. The Yorkshire Dales National Park also has many fine walks, both long and short; the Park publishes leaflets describing the walks and giving a very good introduction to the history and ecology of the area. Write or visit the Park Information Officer (address on page 221).

Another good walk, and one that would fit in well with one of the bike routes from York, is the Wolds Way, sixty-seven miles from Filey Brigg on the Yorkshire coast, south through Thixendale in the Wolds, to North Ferriby on the Humber. This route takes you through pleasant cultivated land and past the "lost villages" of the East Riding—villages abandoned with the advent of intensive sheep farming, which are now being excavated.

NINE
Scotland—The Lowlands

Gin a body meet a body
Coming through the rye;
Gin a body kiss a body,
Need a body cry?

ROBERT BURNS: Coming through the Rye

The Lowlands of Scotland include scenery that is definitely Highland in nature; even parts of the Border Country can be wild, rugged and desolate. To the south of Edinburgh is rolling countryside with the lovely River Tweed cutting through the land. To the north the land assumes the Highland character again, especially around Lochs Lomond and Katrine.

The bike tour of the Lowlands is long: 450 miles. It goes through some very rugged country in the north and could take up to two weeks to complete if the whole length is tackled. In the south you will pass through towns and villages associated with the poet Robert Burns, the author Sir Walter Scott, and that most romantic of historical personages: Mary, Queen of Scots. The route is a south-north-south loop route from Dumfries in the south through Glasgow and by Loch Lomond to the northern point of the tour; then east and south through Perth, Edinburgh and Berwick-upon-Tweed. It is possible to continue north from Loch Lomond into the Highlands. If you do this, and tour the Highlands, you can rejoin the Lowlands tour "in step" as you come down the east side of the Highlands. (See *Biking* in Chapter Ten). This Lowland biking tour begins in the south just north of the end of the Lake District bike tour (See Chapter Eight); and it ends at Berwick-upon-Tweed from where another bike tour going south begins (see Chapter Eight). So the Lowland bike tour may either be taken as an entity in itself, or as a linking route between the North of England and the Highlands of Scotland.

Hiking in the Lowlands can also be a rugged venture. Rights of way are not well defined and there are no official long distance paths as yet such as exist in England. However, there are some old

Roman roads such as the twenty-one mile stretch of the Dere Street from Rochester to Jedburgh and also mountain and hill tracks to the south of Edinburgh.

The bike routes in the Lowlands of Scotland are covered by maps 6 and 7 in the Ordnance Survey Quarter-Inch Series, and by maps 38, 40, 44, 45, 46 and 48 in the Bartholomew 1:100,000 Series.

BIKING

LOWLAND TOUR
(450 miles)

Dumfries to Glasgow (80 miles)

Dumfries (LC) is a sturdy town on the River Nith where the poet Robert Burns spent the last five years of his life, his favourite pub was the Globe Inn and he is buried in a mausoleum in St Michael's Churchyard. Burns, who was born in 1759 and died in 1796, is Scotland's most famous bard. He it is we can all thank for *Auld Lang Syne* and other verses, many written in dialect. His last years were spent as a tax collector after failing at small-time farming.

From Dumfries head north on the A76 and after some four miles you will pass by Ellisland to the right of the main road. A detour is worthwhile for it is here that you can see the farmhouse that Burns built with his own hands on the farm he leased in 1788. He tried to introduce improved farming methods but failed, auctioned off his stock and crops and moved to Dumfries.

Continue north on the A76 for a further four miles then turn left on to a minor road towards Dunscore, turn right after a mile on to another minor road for Penpoint (L). Stay on this minor road north through Penpoint and along the River Nith to Kirconnel where you join the A76 and turn left for Cumnock (C). Turn right in Cumnock on to the A70 to Muirkirk. At Muirkirk turn left on to the A723, and after eight miles turn left on to the B745 to Drumclog. From here turn right on to the A71 and proceed north-east for two miles until you come to a left turning, north, a minor road toward Auldhouse five miles distant. At Auldhouse there is a fork in the road; here you can either fork right to Hamilton where you can catch a train and thereby forego the torture of pedalling through the city of Glasgow, or fork left to Eaglesham where you turn right to go straight into Glasgow (HL) on the A727. The best thing about this city is its nineteenth century architecture, but that is rapidly being destroyed due to the process of urban renewal.

Glasgow to Crianlarich (70 miles)

Go north on Springburn Road in Glasgow on to the A803 and out of the city. Cross the Forth and Clyde Canal and bear left on the A807 to Torrance, where you take the B822 north to the A891, where you turn left for Lennoxtown. From here continue north on the B822 through Fintry (H) and Kipper to Thornhill and stay on the B822 to join the A81 into Callander (LC), a nice little town, often called the gateway to the Highlands. The scenery in the northern part of this Lowland route is very like the true Highland scenery in the far north. Go west from Callander through Brig O'Turk (H) to Trossachs Pier on Loch Katrine. This mountainous area is called the Trossachs and has the classical Scottish scenery with rugged mountains and lakes. Loch Katrine is a beautiful little lake, the setting of Sir Walter Scott's *Lady of the Lake*.

From Trossachs Pier follow a private road around the north shore of the loch to Stronachlacher Pier, and bear west from there on a minor road for Inversnaid on Loch Lomond. This is the largest and one of the loveliest inland waters in Britain. From Inversnaid you can take a ferry across Loch Lomond to Tarbet (C, two miles north) where you proceed north on the A82 along the shore of the loch through Ardlui to Crianlarich (H).

Crianlarich to Blairgowrie (65 miles)

At Crianlarich, bikers continuing north to the Highlands and Islands (see Chapter Ten), should branch left, north, on the A82. But bikers who are staying in the Lowlands will bear right, north-east, on the A85 along the River Dochart to Killin (HCL) where there is a prehistoric circle of standing stones; nearby is Loch Tay. Bear left at Killin on to the A827 going along the north shore of the loch to Kenmore (L), which is a pretty little village: you can visit the inn where Robert Burns left an inscription over the fireplace in the parlour. From Kenmore bear north-east on the A827 through Aberfeldy (HCL), a quiet little market town situated in lovely countryside. Continue along the A827 to Grandtully where you bear right on to a minor road into Inver, and then on to the A9 north for one mile, then right on to the A923 to Blairgowrie (L), a town set in the midst of the raspberry farms. (The route coming south from the Highlands and Islands connects here, see Chapter Ten.)

Blairgowrie to Stirling (85 miles)

Continue south on the A93; after a few miles you will pass through Meiklour where there is, along the roadside, an immense 230 year old beech hedge, almost one hundred feet high and six hundred yards long. Follow the A93 south through Cargill (C) into Perth (HLC) a city of about fifty thousand people and for many years the capital of Scotland. Take the A90 south and turn left on to the A912. Stay on this road until it meets the A91 where you turn left. After a couple of miles, turn right on to the A983 going south for Falkland (H), a little cobbled town. Here you can see Falkland Palace, a favourite of the royal house of Stuart, and a retreat for one of the Stuart's most famous representatives: Mary, Queen of Scots. From Falkland bear right on a minor road over the Lomond Hills to Leslie on the A911, on which you turn right, west, to Milnathort, where you bear left, south, down to Kinross (C) on Loch Leven. Mary Queen of Scots was imprisoned for a time in the castle in the middle of Loch Leven. From Kinross go south on the B996 to Cowdenbeath where you bear right to go through Dunfermline, capital of Scotland long ago, and now a large textile centre. Andrew Carnegie, the famous industrialist, was born here. He gave a fine park to the town and the cottage where he was born is now a museum. Take the A994 west out of Dunfermline across the A985 to Torryburn, and then right on a minor road parallel to the A985 to Culross, probably the most complete example of a medieval village, or burgh, in Scotland. Continue west to Kincardine, and then north on the A977; turn left on to the A907 through Alloa (C) to the A91 where you turn left for Stirling (HCL), an attractive little university town with a beautiful castle high on a rock overlooking the town. Mary Queen of Scots was crowned at this castle when she was six days old, her father having died shortly before her birth. There is a music festival held here in mid-May.

Stirling to Edinburgh (40 miles)

Head south-east on the A905 through Grangemouth to Bowness where you turn right on the A706 to Linlithgow. From Linlithgow take the B9080 east. Just before Edinburgh the B9080 joins the A8 which takes you into the centre of the city.

Edinburgh (HLC) is another of those fantastic but strangely

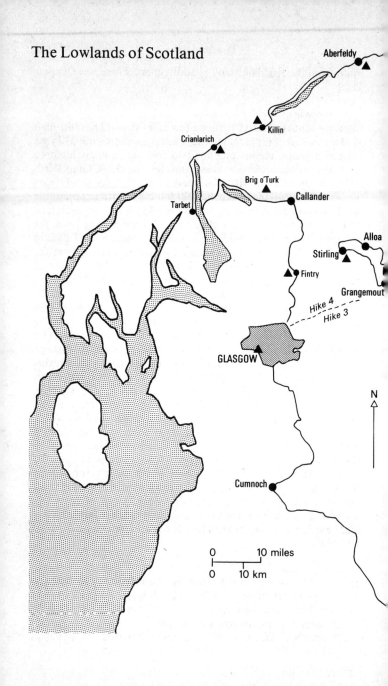

The Lowlands of Scotland

Aberfeldy

Killin

Crianlarich

Brig o'Turk

Callander

Tarbet

Alloa

Stirling

Fintry

Grangemout

Hike 4

Hike 3

GLASGOW

Cumnoch

N

0   10 miles
0   10 km

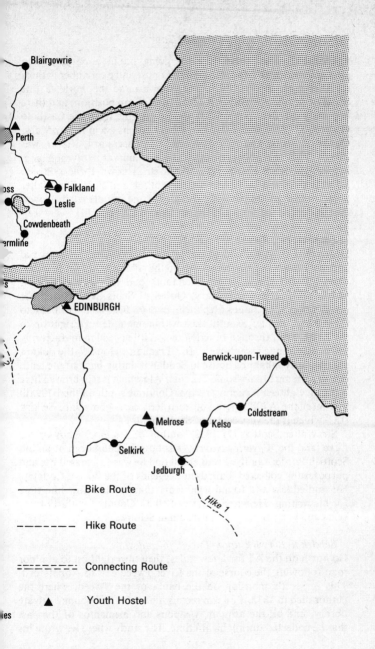

Blairgowrie

Perth

ss
Falkland
Leslie
Cowdenbeath
rmline

s

EDINBURGH

Berwick-upon-Tweed

Coldstream
Melrose
Kelso
Selkirk
Jedburgh
Hike 1

—————— Bike Route

— — — — — Hike Route

======== Connecting Route

▲ Youth Hostel

ies

under-rated cities; there is a lot going on in a cosmopolitan atmosphere: an arts festival in mid-August and September gathers together great theatre and music from around the world, a fine castle overlooks the entire city from its hill-top position, and there are many excellent pubs. Walk the Royal Mile from the Castle to Holyrood Palace where you can see the rooms occupied by Mary, Queen of Scots, and the room where her secretary, Rizzio, was killed. Visit the abbey ruins in the grounds at Holyrood and, before you leave Edinburgh, take a stroll down Princes Street. Edinburgh is the birthplace of the author and poet, Sir Walter Scott, whose monument sits proudly in the middle of the town. (See under *Hiking* for walks in and around Edinburgh.)

Edinburgh to Selkirk (50 miles)

Head south from Edinburgh on the A68 to Dalkeith, an industrial and market town. Continue south on the A7 for about seven miles. Turn left off the A7 down a minor road to the east to visit Borthwick Castle where Mary, Queen of Scots lived during her honeymoon with James Hepburn, Earl of Bothwell. Go back to the A7 and turn left, south, then within one mile turn right on to the B709, west, through Innerleithen, a little tweed manufacturing town. Continue south-west to Traquair House, the oldest continuously inhabited house in Scotland, dating back to the tenth century. Be sure to try some Traquair Ale which is still brewed here using an eighteenth century recipe. Continue south on the B709 till you meet the A708 where you turn left, east, going into Selkirk (LC) which is the very centre of Scott country.

Sir Walter Scott (1771-1832), author of *Ivanhoe, Lady of the Lake,* and the *Waverley Novels,* was born in Edinburgh of an old Scottish Border family. From childhood he was fascinated by, and purposefully collected, ballads and legends of the Border Country. He studied law and found legal work that would allow him time for his writing. He was Sheriff of Selkirk County for thirty-three years and you can see his courtroom in Selkirk.

Selkirk to Berwick-upon-Tweed, (60 miles)

Go north on the A7 for a few miles, then turn right on to a minor road following the course of the River Tweed east to Abbotsford. This is Scott's mansion on the banks of the Tweed, where the author died in 1832. You can see his nine thousand volume private library, and all the armour, weapons and mementos of the past that he collected during his lifetime. The study where he wrote his novels is preserved as Scott left it.

Continue north-east to the A6091 where you turn right for Melrose (HLC), a little town that grew up beside a seventh century abbey, one of a series of so-called "Border Abbeys". The ruins of Melrose, mostly from the fifteenth century, are glorious to see—especially the window tracery of the south transept. A few miles south-east is Dryburgh Abbey. Proceed south on the A6091 and just after this road merges with the A68, you will see signs to Dryburgh, just to the east of the A68. This is another of the beautiful Border Abbeys, it is over eight hundred years old and Sir Walter Scott is buried here.

Go back to the A68 and south into Jedburgh (C) (see under *Hiking*), another village which grew up around a beautiful abbey. Scott made his first appearance as a lawyer in the court-house at Jedburgh, successfully pleading for a poacher; and, at the Mary Queen of Scots House, you can see Mary's death-mask. It was from Jedburgh that Mary rode one night, before their marriage, to see Bothwell who had been wounded while catching an outlaw. This night ride back and forth covered some twenty miles across dangerous country—especially dangerous for an unescorted lady and especially the Queen of Scotland. Upon her return from this adventure, the Queen fell into a fever and it is said that Bothwell had his litter brought to Jedburgh and the two recovered together.

From Jedburgh, go back north on the A68 turning right on to the A698 to go through Kelso (CL), a beautiful little town with the remains of a twelfth century abbey. Continue on the A698 east to the A697 and bear right into Coldstream (C) on the River Tweed. This was once a refuge for eloping couples: at one time it was possible in Scotland to be married merely by making a solemn statement in front of witnesses. Head east on the A697 out of Coldstream and then turn left on to the A698 again for Berwick-upon-Tweed (LC) and the end of the tour. From this point you can rejoin the routes going south (see Chapter Eight).

HIKING

There are no official long distance paths in Scotland. There is one in the planning stage called the West Highlands Way, from Glasgow north to Fort William; but it will probably be several years before right of way agreements are worked out. It can be hard and lonely walking here and even more so farther north. It is best to have camping equipment, a good supply of maps and knowledge of navigation skills before setting out on your own.

DERE STREET ROMAN ROAD
(21 miles)

Half of this hike really belongs in the North of England, but as it finishes in the Scottish Border Country I have included it in this chapter. The route follows an old Roman road called Dere Street, constructed in the second century AD. On this stretch of Dere Street you will discover the fallacy that Roman roads are always straight. Roman engineers, it is true, did prefer a straight line, but were not unwilling to use a winding road where it was needed on hilly ground. These Roman roads have lasted so long because they were so well constructed with a layer of large stones a foot deep, covered by a further four inches of small stones, and on top of this a binding of clay. The roads were sided with large stones along the whole length. Many Roman roads were more than twenty feet wide.

Useful maps for this route are the Ordnance Survey 1:50,000 Series, numbers 74 and 80. Accommodation along the track is difficult to find so carry camping equipment, and as always, good hiking boots and rain gear are needed. The path in the Roxburgh County section of Scotland has been waymarked by the county council.

1. *Rochester to Jedburgh (21 miles)*

Dere Street begins at Rochester (L), five miles north of Otterburn. *(As part of the road north of here runs across artillery ranges, make enquiries at the Redesdale Camp before you set out as to when firing will take place.)* Follow the road, a broad track, north to Bremenium, then a straight three miles to Featherwood, then along a paved road by Outer Golden Pot and north-west again on the track to the large Roman camp at Chew Green. (This marks the end of the firing ranges.) From here it is one mile north to the Scottish border, over the Cheviots at Black Halls, and then Blackhall Hill and north-west to cross the Kale Water to Tow Ford. North of here you go by Whitton Edge and Shibden Hill, and by Cappuck (a Roman fort) to the east of Jedburgh (C), and on up to the bridge over the Jed Water at Jedfoot, two miles north of Jedburgh.

HILL WALKING NEAR EDINBURGH

You can have a pleasant few hours of walking during your visit to Edinburgh by taking the bus from the city to Hillend and walking up past the artificial ski slope at Caerketton. There are fine views from here across the city of Edinburgh and the Firth of Forth. You can continue the walk on to Allermuir and from there down to the village of Swanston.

2. *The Pentland Hills*

There are also some fine walks in the Pentland Hills to the south of Edinburgh. These walks begin at various places along the Edinburgh/West Linton Road (A702) and cross the Pentlands to the north-west to end at, or just south-west of, the village of Balerno on the A70 road. The walks are well sign-posted along the paths and at the entrance and exit points. There is also a good hill walk in the Pentlands running parallel to the A702 between Glencorse and Nine Mile Barn. This path leads over Carneth Hill, Scald Law, East Kip, and West Kip. These routes are from five to seven miles in length. Another good route of nine miles leads from Carlops on the A702 to Balerno on the A70.

Carry the Ordnance Survey 1:50,000 Series map number 66 for these routes, or the Bartholomew 1:100,000 Series map number 41.

OTHER WALKS IN THE LOWLANDS

3. *The Antonine Wall*

The Antonine Wall, originally stretching for thirty-six miles between the Firth of Forth and Firth of Clyde, was built twenty years after Hadrian's Wall. Built mostly of turf, it was constructed after a re-conquest of the Lowlands; some of the best preserved sections which also provide good walks are between Rough Castle and Westerwood.

4. *The Forth and Clyde Canal*

The Forth and Clyde Canal, an old industrial canal which has now fallen into disuse runs between the Clyde and the Forth to the north of the Antonine Wall, from Bowling Basin on the north bank of the Clyde, through Glasgow, Kirkintilloch, Kilsyth, Bonnybridge, and Falkirk, to Grangemouth Docks on the Forth. There are good walks on the tow path along most stretches of the canal; the best parts are in the Bowling, Kilsyth, and Falkirk areas.

An excellent guide covering hikes and walks in the Lowlands is: *Scotland for Hillwalking,* published by the Scottish Tourist Board and available from any of the many tourist offices in Scotland. Another invaluable source of routes for walkers is the *Scottish Hill Tracks—Old Highways and Drove Roads—Southern Scotland,* by D. G. Moir. This pamphlet is available from Bartholomew and Sons on Duncan Street in Edinburgh. It contains over 150 well described routes with maps included.

TEN

Scotland—
The Highlands
and Islands

*Sir, the noblest prospect that a Scotchman ever
sees is the high road that leads him to London.*

SAMUEL JOHNSON: Tour of the Hebrides

Such a slanderous remark from Dr Johnson may have seemed true
in his day—now, I venture to say, it is the other way round. With
the natural landscape being everywhere swallowed up as human
populations increase, Scotland has become a haven: the Highlands
and Islands are the out-back of Europe, very rugged country and
usually quite desolate. Yet there are places in the Highlands that
boast a tourist industry as lively as in Cornwall. But in many parts
of the Highlands you will not even see a goat, let alone another
human being. Much of northern Scotland, especially on the
Islands, is Gaelic speaking. Those who speak Gaelic usually speak
English too, but the place-names are mostly of Gaelic derivation,
so knowing a few Gaelic words could make your travels more
interesting:

aber: mouth or confluence
　　of a river
ben, beann, beinn: mountain
caolas: a strait or firth
car: a bend, winding
coire, corrie: hollow
dubh, dhu: black, dark
dun: hill fort
eilean: island

inch, innis: island
inver, inbhir: mouth of a river
mor, more: great, extensive
ross: forest, peninsula
ru, rhu, row, rudha: point
strath: broad valley
tobar: well
uamh: cave
uig: sheltered bay or nook

In the Highlands, battles, famous people and old churches seem unimportant beside the vastness and grandeur of nature; the traces of man seem very insignificant in comparison with the mountains, the mysterious lochs, the heaths and the long summer days when the sun hardly sets.

There is one colossal bike route which connects in the West with the Lowlands bike route at Crianlarich and loops up north through the Highlands and Islands for almost a thousand miles to meet the Lowlands bike tour, going south, in East Scotland, at Blairgowrie. The distances are so vast that this route could easily take a month—of *steady* biking. I would not advise anyone but the very fit and the fanatical to attempt the whole thing. The biking is hard in the Highlands, with many steep gradients, changeable weather, and long distances to pedal between towns just to find a night's lodging. However, if you utilize the railway, you can pick and choose stretches of the route that you, in particular, wish to bike. For example, there is a two week tour which you can begin at Glen Coe or Fort William in the west, then go north out to the islands of Skye and the Outer Hebrides, return by ferry to Ullapool, then continue east across the Highlands to Inverness to link up with the trains going south. But there are many other options and some may even want to do the whole thousand-mile route.

Hiking in the Highlands can also be a rugged affair. I have provided a few day-long walks and two climbs, but no long, cross-country hikes. Official long distance routes do not exist yet in Scotland, and the shorter walks given here are fairly easy to follow and not too rugged. Hill-walking and long distance hiking in Scotland should not be attempted by any but those who are in good physical condition, who enjoy camping out, who are competent in the use of compass and map, and who know the common safety measures which must be observed in isolated mountain areas.

There are not many official B and Bs in Scotland (especially in the Islands), though private homes will sometimes take in travellers. These homes do not, however, usually have a sign indicating that you can lodge there, so it is sensible to use the Scottish system of "Book a Bed Ahead": at any of the main villages you will find a small tourist office, and, for a minimal charge, the people there will reserve you a place in the next town or village. This is especially important in the Islands which are somewhat raw and primitive even today. Another helpful hint: Scotland's postal system runs a mini-bus service every day to collect and deliver mail along the rural backroads; there are some fifty routes throughout the country, with an outward journey in the morning and a homeward journey after lunch. The mini-buses take a limited number of passengers and you can get a timetable from any Post Office in Scotland. These buses will take you to remote parts of the country, which, without a car, you would never have time to see. You may want to ride out in the morning, take a walk or picnic in the remote countryside, then catch the red mini-bus on its way back in the afternoon.

The bike routes in the Highlands of Scotland are covered by maps 1, 2, 3, 4 and 5 in the Ordnance Survey Quarter-Inch Series, and by maps 47, 48, 49, 50, 51, 52, 54, 55, 58, 59 and 60 (Outer Hebrides: 53 and 57, Orkney and Shetland: 61 and 62) in the Bartholomew 1:100,000 Series.

BIKING

HIGHLANDS and ISLANDS
(945 miles)

This is not for the timid or weak-thighed. The whole route could easily take a month, but the best part, to my mind, is in the west and the Outer Hebrides. There are connections in the west and east with the bike route for the Lowlands.

Crianlarich to Mallaig (100 miles)
From Crianlarich (H), the northern point of the Lowlands bike tour, take the A82 north through the Bridge of Orchy over fairly mountainous terrain with typical Highland scenery. Stay on the A82 into Glen Coe—a forbidding place on a rainy day, but lovely and crisp on a sunny day, with high mountains towering over the road and waterfalls cascading to right and left. Continue west on the A82 to Glencoe town (HLC), west on the A828 to Ballachulish to catch a ferry across Loch Leven, and on to the A82 again north to Fort William (LCH three miles away at Glen Nevis, see under *Hiking*). This, despite its military-sounding name, is a surprisingly pretty little town which lies at the foot of Ben Nevis; it is also an important tourist centre. Ben Nevis (see under *Hiking*), at 4400 feet, is the highest mountain in Britain and is well worth climbing

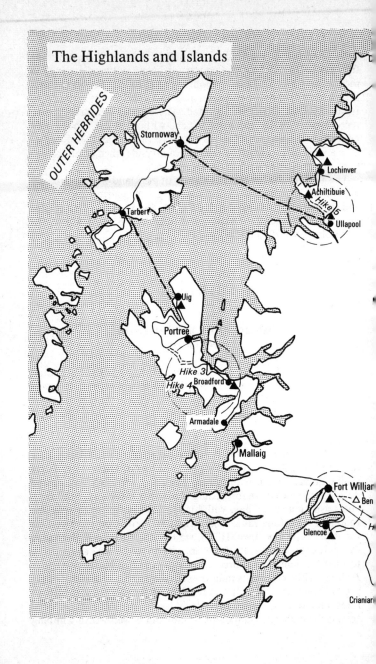

The Highlands and Islands

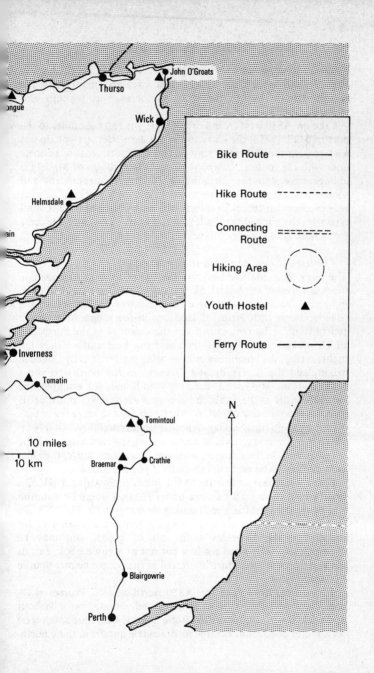

by one of its easier paths. There are some good wool craft shops in Fort William which sell fine, warm sweaters, many with the natural lanolin left in the wool to increase its warmth and protective qualities.

Take the A830 west from Fort William for forty-six miles to the port of Mallaig (L), the entry to the Western Isles. (If you do not wish to visit the Hebrides, stay on the A82 north-east to connect later with the route at Ullapool.) The fishing village of Mallaig is unimpressive, but the surrounding country is magnificent and somewhat awesome. *Johnson's,* a fishing supply store on the pier, sells excellent turtleneck sweaters—the heavy black and white wool type with the natural lanolin left in the wool. You catch the ferry from Mallaig to the Isle of Skye.

The Isle of Skye: Armadale to Uig (85 miles)

The ferry from Mallaig lands on the Isle of Skye at Armadale in the south-west of the Island. Skye is one of the less remote islands, but many features you see here also hold true for the rest of the islands. These little strips of land out in the rough Atlantic are generally quite barren, except for the Orkneys to the north-east which make much of their income from beef cattle. They are highly ethnic, the Hebridean culture being predominantly Gaelic in origin, and the Shetlands and Orkneys in the north-east more Scandinavian. The islands are very traditional; for example, the Sabbath really is the Sabbath here, and even public transport is shut down on the day of rest, so when you want to leave the islands do not try to go on a Sunday. Another island speciality, notably on Skye, are the midges which come out in the mornings and the evenings and, in the summer, wherever there is moisture; they bite unmercifully so be warned, especially if you are camping.

From Armadale follow the A851 north to Broadford (HL), a small island town on a bay (see under *Hiking*) where Dr Johnson and Boswell stayed for a spell during their trip to Skye in 1773. By the way, if you are thinking of using Johnson's journal of his journey to the Hebrides as a sort of guide, you may be disappointed—it is good reading but not as a guide book, for, as always, Johnson was more interested in the people he met than in the countryside.

From Broadford take the A850 north-west to Portree (LC), considered to be the capital of the island, situated on a harbour and packed with white-washed stone houses. Continue south-west on a minor road from Portree to Bracadale and from there north-west on the A863 to Dunvegan (LC), which has one of the oldest inhabited castles in the country, said to date from the ninth century. This is the ancestral home of the MacLeods, a clan that figures prominently in the history of the island. Bear right on the A850 to Carbost then left on to a minor road to Kensaleyne on the A856 and north to Uig (HCL), which is a pleasant conglomeration of crofts, or small land-holdings, and cottages on a hillside overlooking a harbour; you can catch the ferry from here to Tarbert on the island of Harris in the Outer Hebrides. The trip takes about two hours.

The Outer Hebrides: Tarbert to Stornaway (140 miles)

Harris is the southern portion of the Isle of Lewis—the Outer Hebrides also encompasses the Uists to the south. Tarbert (L), where you land from the ferry, is a peninsula connecting South Harris with the rest of the island. These islands are the home of Harris Tweed and still the centre of the Harris tweed industry. The tweed is made from Scottish wool by about twelve hundred cottage workers in the Outer Hebrides; the wool is spun and dyed and hand-woven by the islanders. There are over seven million yards of tweed woven per year in over five thousand different colours and designs; you can buy a hand-tailored suit from a small tailor's shop for a very reasonable price; and, best of all, you can see the material being made from start to finish.

Go south from Tarbert on the A859. You will find some good, deserted beaches. Continue south to Leverburgh, named after Lord Leverhulme who once owned the island and tried unsuccessfully to improve its economy by backing the fish trade. Continue south to Rodel, and then turn north on a minor road through Manish to the A859, back through Tarbert and north into mountainous and rugged terrain; then, through Balallan, into the flats of Lewis. Stay on the A859 through Laxay (L) for a further six miles, then turn left on to a minor road through Achmore, on to the A858 and to the stone circle at Callanish. This stone circle ranks with Stonehenge: its isolated setting and the jagged shape of the standing stones give it a real sense of Bronze Age mystery, and it is distinctly spooky!

Proceed north on the A858 through Carloway (L) to Arnol where some of the old traditional homes of the islanders—so called "black houses"—have been turned into museums and can be visited. The name of these low-built stone dwellings probably derives from the fact that they had no chimneys to allow the smoke from the ever-present peat fire to escape. Bear right at Barvas on to the A857 into Stornaway (LC), a centre for Harris Tweed, and the only place in the Outer Hebrides large enough to be called a town. You can catch the ferry from here to Ullapool on the mainland: a three-hour trip.

Ullapool to Thurso (170 miles)

Ullapool (LCH), a little fishing village—both commercial and game—is situated in a lovely corner of the county of Ross and Cromarty (see under *Hiking*).

Take the A835 north from Ullapool for nine miles then turn left on to a minor road along Loch Lurgainn; bear right after about seven miles on to another minor road going north through Inverkirkaig (CH), through Stoer (H) and Drumbeg; then back on to the A894 on which you turn left, north, and encounter some ten miles of rough going over steep gradients. The A894 merges with the A838 and continues north to Durness (LH), then south along Loch Eriboll into some more hilly biking. Follow the A838 along the north coast to Tongue (LCH): the tidal estuary here is excellent bird-watching territory where many varieties of sea birds gather (see under *Hiking*).

Continue east on the A836 through Strathy and past the nuclear power station at Dounreay to Thurso (LC). This is an old Viking settlement—its name comes from the Norse and means "Thor's River"; the town is situated on a river rich in salmon and trout, and there are the ruins of a seventeenth century castle, home of the Earls of Sinclair, above the harbour. The town has grown greatly since the advent of the nearby nuclear plant but the growth has been fairly well planned. The ferry to Stromness in the Orkneys leaves from Scrabster just north-east of Thurso. It is a two and a half hour trip. If you do not wish to visit the Orkneys and Shetland Islands, proceed east on the A836 from Thurso on the next stretch of the mainland route.

The Orkney and Shetland Islands: Stromness via Lerwick to Stromness (150 miles)

You land on the island of the Orkney cluster known as the Mainland. It is beef cattle and egg country, low-lying with only a few hills. The Orkneys and Shetlands were influenced, both in language and culture, by the Norse who ruled them until the fifteenth century. The islands became part of Britain only in 1468 when they were given as a pledge for the dowry of Margaret, princess of Norway, who was betrothed to James III of Scotland. The pledge was never redeemed and so the islands came under Scottish rule. From the harbour town of Stromness (LCH), where you land on Orkney, travel north on the A967 by the Loch of Stenness to The Barony or Brough Head. Continue around the northern tip of the island on the A967 to Redland then take the A966 south into Finstown. From there take the A965 east into Kirkwall (L) where you can catch a ferry to Lerwick in the Shetland Islands: an eight hour trip.

Lerwick (HL) is the main town of the Shetlands and home to more than half the population of the island. It is a strangely cosmopolitan little town in the midst of the remotest reaches of the British Isles. The hundred islands in the Shetland group are on the same latitude as Greenland and Siberia, but the proximity of the Gulf Stream keeps the climate relatively warm. However, there are raging storms and heavy gales that whip across the flat, treeless moorland landscape of the islands. The Shetlands are weaving country and home of the Shetland sweater. The men make their living mostly from the sea, and now from the North Sea oil industry and the increasing tourist trade as well.

Travel south from Lerwick on the A970 through Fladdabister to the extreme southern tip of the island at Sumburgh (L), where there is an airport. Near here is Jarlshof: a fascinating archaeological site which shows evidence of continuous occupation by various groups from about 1000 BC to AD 1600. Backtrack north and take a minor road looping to the left through Scousburgh, and then back again on to the A970, north through Fladdabister and bear left to go past the airport at Tingwall, then turn left on to the A971 through Tresta. Bear right on a minor road going north through Aith and Voe (L) and back on to the A970, where you bear right, south, back down into Lerwick and the ferry south to the Orkneys at Kirkwall.

From Kirkwall bear left on the A960, then left on a minor road which will connect you with the A961 through St Mary's and back into Kirkwall. From there take the A965 south-east past two fine archaeological sites. The first is at Maes Howe which is a large round cairn, or hollow mound of rocks over a burial, from about 2500 BC. This is the best example of its kind in Britain and has obvious links with cairns in Ireland such as at Newgrange. Next you will come to the Stenness (L) stone circle, a major one of its kind with several stone circles inside a circular ditch. It was probably an important religious site in its day and it must have

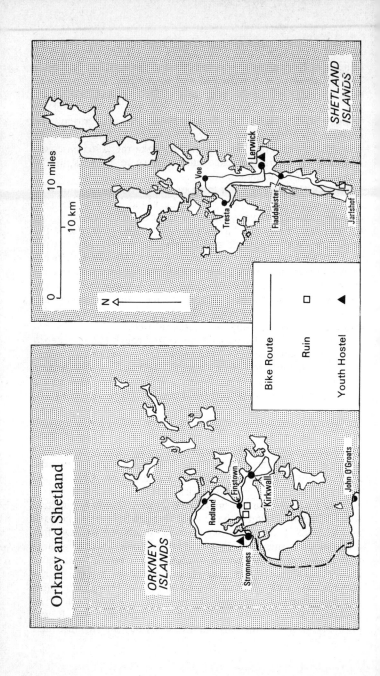

Orkney and Shetland

ORKNEY ISLANDS

Redland
Finstown
Kirkwall
Strommess
John O'Groats

SHETLAND ISLANDS

Voe
Tresta
Lerwick
Haddabister
Jarlshof

N

0   10 km
0   10 miles

Bike Route
□   Ruin
▲   Youth Hostel

been a powerful religion to reach the inhabitants of such a remote area as the Orkneys.

Continue on to Stromness where you take the ferry back to the mainland.

Thurso to Inverness (160 miles)

Travel east on the A836 from Thurso to Dunnet (L) where you can make a detour on the B855 out to Dunnet Head, the most northerly point of the British mainland, to see the fine cliffs, the lighthouse and the puffins.

Continue east on the A836 to John O'Groats (LCH), a usual goal for Highland bikers; the place was named after a Dutchman, John de Groot, who was a local ferryman. Continue south on the A9 through Wick (LC), an old boom town from the herring-fishing days, which Robert Louis Stevenson once described as "the bleakest of God's towns in the baldest of God's bays". Stay on the A9 south through Helmsdale (HLC), a fishing port famous for lobsters—mostly exported to France, through the little resort town of Brora (LC) to Bonar Bridge (L) where you bear right on to the A836. Stay on the main road until you come to a left turn for Culrain (HC). From Culrain you take a minor road south to the A9 at Ardgay and continue south on that road through Evanton (C) and the workingman's town of Dingwall (LC) into Inverness (HCL). Inverness, which many call the "Capital of the Highlands", is a pleasant little town, but at the height of the season it can be as crowded as Brighton on Bank Holiday; so book ahead if possible for accommodation.

Inverness to Blairgowrie (140 miles)

Take the A862 south-west from Inverness and along Loch Ness, which, at twenty two miles, is the longest Loch in Scotland, it is also very deep. Several people live in tents along the lake hoping to photograph the legendary monster. There have been some quite definitive shots of "Nessie", as she is affectionately called. If it exists, the theory is that "Nessie" must be a sea creature cut off from the ocean waters as the sea receded in distant geological times; the animal, or animals afterwards evolved alone—separated from the rest of the species which probably became extinct, as did the plesiosaurs which this animal is supposed to resemble. Pictures show Nessie to be long-necked with a hump-like body, very reminiscent of the age of dinosaurs: so what some observers believe to exist in Loch Ness is an evolutionary freak—an ancient species saved from extinction by being captured in an alien but compatible environment.

Follow a minor road along the loch from Dores, bear left on a minor road through Errogie and travel north on the A862; then bear right on a minor road through Croachy, then right again on a minor road and left on another for Tomatin on the A9. Travel south on the A9 and bear left at Carrbridge on to the A938 to Dulnain Bridge (L) in the Spey Valley. This is popular mountaineering country and also ski country in the winter with many Swiss-style resorts. Go south on the A95 to a turning to the left on a minor road through Nethy Bridge to the A939 where you turn right. You will come to some fine scenery here but also to some tough biking country as you go over the Grampian Mountains. Go through Tomintaul (LCH) and continue south on the A939 until you come to a turning to the right on to a minor road for Crathie on the A93. Bear right at Crathie to Braemar (H) where there is a Royal Highland Gathering in September.

Stay on the A93 south to Blairgowrie (L) where you meet the Lowland Biking tour going south (see Chapter Nine).

HIKING

Hiking in the Highlands and Islands, as in the Lowlands, can be a rugged affair; the waymarked paths that are so omnipresent down south, are anomalies here, and weather, as well as rights of way, can play havoc with your plans. Carry an extra pair of trousers, stout boots and a good waterproof. Know how to read a map before you tackle the hills and do not overdo it: Scotland is an unforgiving country and not even God protects fools. Know the basics of compass navigation and check with wardens at the various hostels to confirm your routes and to get some last minute tips. Remember that even the easiest routes can be treacherous when the mists set in suddenly.

Two good publications are: *Scotland for Hillwalking* published by the Scottish Tourist Board and available from any of the tourist offices in Scotland; and *Scottish Hill Tracks and Drove Roads—Northern Scotland,* by D. G. Moir, published by Bartholomew in Edinburgh.

A WALK AND A CLIMB AROUND FORT WILLIAM

1. *Ben Nevis Climb*

This mountain looms at 4406 feet over Fort William. There is a fairly easy and well-marked ascent. You should be in good physical condition for the climb, and be prepared for any weather: the mists blow in very quickly in the Scottish mountains. Stay on the path.

Starting from the hostel at Glen Nevis cross the river and climb directly upwards to join a well-made path that zig-zags up to the boulder-strewn plateau at the summit. There is generally snow on Ben Nevis until summer and care should be taken when approaching edges at the summit plateau, for there may be huge and unstable snow cornices. Allow four to five hours for the ascent and about three hours for the descent. Start early to give yourself plenty of daylight hours for the climb. Another path around the north-east side of Ben Nevis gives you better views, but it is also more difficult and should not be attempted without good maps and detailed instructions about the correct paths to follow. Ben Nevis should be climbed only in good, clear weather.

2. *Kinlochleven to Fort William (15 miles)*

There is an old military road between these two points that provides a good day's walk on an easy-to-follow track. The military road begins on the north side of Kinlochleven, zig-zags up the hillside to the north and proceeds west above the Allt Nathrac. From here the road goes through a pass, then by Lairigmor and down the Alt na Lairige Moire to Blarmchfodach and into Fort William. The last five miles are on surfaced road.

Carry map number 41 in the Ordnance Survey 1:50,000 Series for these routes.

WALKING ON THE ISLE OF SKYE

3. *Broadford Circular Walk*

From Broadford (LH) there is a pleasant day's outing that follows the shoreline. It is easy to follow: just keep the sea on your left. There is plenty of opportunity for exploring tidal pools along the rocky shoreline. The walk can be difficult in wet weather because of the rocky nature of the coastline and the slippery surfaces. There are no impassable stretches, just the inconvenience of crossing the jagged rocks.

Proceed north out of Broadford village on to the A850 also called the New Road, toward Portree. You will soon find that the Old Road runs parallel to this new one, and that you can walk on it rather than on the noisy road now used. Keep going north on one of these roads—they are always in sight of one another—for about three miles, to just past the cemetery on the right, where you will find a turnstile gate that leads you through forestry land and down to the seashore. From here just make your way around the shore and back into Broadford. Watch out for the midges at points along the walk where there is swampy ground.

No map is needed for this hike as you will either be on roads or following the line of the coast.

4. *The Cuillins*

The Isle of Skye is noted for the Cuillins, the mountain range in the south-west, which is undoubtedly the most difficult and savage range in the whole of the British Isles; they are the steepest and rockiest mountains you will find in Britain and they are not for the beginner. You will not be able to reach the top of the range without a good knowledge of rock climbing, but if you are an experienced rock climber you may enjoy the challenge. The Scottish Mountaineering Club publishes a detailed description in its *Isle of Skye* handbook; the Glen Brittle Hostel provides the best point of access to the range. The peaks are not high, averaging around three thousand feet, but they are steep and usually cloud-covered and should be attempted only in fine weather.

A WALK FROM ULLAPOOL

This walk could take up to seven hours to the hostel at Achiltibuie, on a fairly well-marked path along the slopes of a mountain and along cliffs above the sea. In places the path can be difficult and care is needed on the cliffs. Do not attempt the path when the visibility is bad, for posts and rock piles mark the path and you must keep these in sight, especially along the cliffs.

You will need a map for this route: the Ordnance Survey 1:50,000 Series number 19.

5. *Ullapool to Achiltibuie (17 miles)*

From Ullapool follow the A835 north for about five miles and then bear left on to a minor road to South Keanchulish. After a mile you will see a bridge crossing a river where you turn west. A little further on you will come to a wicket gate in a fence and from here the path climbs steeply uphill to about the eight-hundred foot level. From this point on the path is marked by posts and rock piles. Continue along the slope of Ben More Coigach and along the edge of the cliffs. At one point, Culnacraig, you have a choice of routes: you can either branch inland by road to Achiltibuie, or follow the sea by path to Achduart and from there by road to the Achininver Hostel at Achiltibuie.

CLIMBING BEN LOYAL

6. *Climbing Ben Loyal*

Ben Loyal to the south of Tongue is not the most challenging climb in Scotland, but it can provide a good day's hill-walking. Your best starting point for the ascent of Ben Loyal is Ribigill Farm, two miles south of Tongue (HL). From here a good track leads across the moor towards the steep peak of Chaonasaid. Head south-east below the foot of this peak to reach easier grassy slopes beyond; from here it is a fairly easy climb south-west to reach the summit of Ben Loyal. Chaonsaid is the northern terminus of the summit and the highest peak, A'Chaistael (2500 feet) is half a mile to the south.

The east side of Ben Loyal is moorland and easy to climb, but rather dull. Begin this ascent from Loch Loyal. The west side is very steep.

Check with the warden at the Tongue Hostel for further advice on routes and up-to-date tips. Only attempt the climb in good weather. You will need the Ordnance Survey map in the 1:50,000 Series, number 10.

ELEVEN
East Anglia and The Fens

For England's the one land, I know,
Where men with Splendid Hearts may go,
And Cambridgeshire, of all England,
The shire for Men who Understand.

RUPERT BROOKE: The Old Vicarage, Grantchester

The poet, Rupert Brooke, may have been biased but his bias has more than a grain of truth in it: this last touring area has something for everyone. Not the rugged, lonely beauty of the north, but a peaceful, gently flowing landscape that rivals the north with a contrasting sort of beauty. East Anglia and the Fens is a marvellous area for biking: the landscape is flat and gentle enough even to require dykes to protect the land from the sea. It is a strange mixture of busy seaside resorts on the coastline near Norwich, and undiscovered villages inland.

The bike tour includes several fine cathedral cities as well as the university town of Cambridge, and it passes through many lovely little villages which still retain their medieval flavour. Towards the south-east end of the tour there is a mini-tour of places associated with the painter John Constable. And linking the whole 265 miles together is a string of pubs: the best pubs that East Anglia has to offer. For hikers, there are sections of two Roman roads where you can stretch your legs and marvel at the skill of the Roman engineers.

The bike routes in East Anglia and The Fens are covered by maps 11 and 14 in the Ordnance Survey Quarter-Inch Series, and by maps 5, 6, 8, 9 and 10 in the Bartholomew 1:100,000 Series.

BIKING

CATHEDRALS, COLLEGES, CONSTABLE and PUBS
(265 miles)

Lincoln to Peterborough (75 miles)

Lincoln (LH) has the third largest cathedral in England, dating from the thirteenth century; it looks much like Canterbury Cathedral, with a magnificent tower, 271 feet high. This is one of the four great cathedral cities in Lincolnshire and East Anglia: Ely, Peterborough and Norwich being the other three. The town of Lincoln, which began existence as a Roman military garrison, stands at the junction of several Roman roads.

Head south from Lincoln on a minor road through Branston and Digby, bearing right on to the A153 into Sleaford. Take the A17 to the east out of Sleaford and then bear left on to the A1121 for Boston. In the middle ages Boston, as a port, was second only to London, though today the waters have receded. See the Boston Stump, one of the largest parish churches in England, with superb views from the tower. The Stump is actually a metaphorical timepiece: the church has seven doors, there are twelve pillars in the nave, twenty-four steps to the library, fifty-two windows, sixty steps to the chancel roof, and 365 steps up to the top of the tower.

From Boston take the A16 south to Spalding. There is a tulip festival held here in May. This Riding of Lincolnshire is called Holland and the dykes holding back the North Sea should complete a picture of a little Holland in your mind. Take the A1073 south from Spalding, and then bear right on to the A47 into Peterborough (LC) three miles to the west: this is a large market town with a fine Guildhall; the cathedral dates from the twelfth century and is in the Romanesque style, a facade in the early Gothic style now covers the old Romanesque west front.

Peterborough to Cambridge (85 miles)

From Peterborough head east on the A605 and then bear right on to a minor road into March, formerly the capital of the Isle of Ely. The church has a fine hammerbeam roof dating from the fifteenth century, carved with nearly two hundred angels. Try the White Horse Inn on Darthill Road—it has a pleasant garden.

Take the A141 south from March to Chatteris where the Ye Old George Hotel on the High Street is a fine two hundred year old pub which serves good mutton and prawns in the dining room; Chatteris is one of the oldest towns in the Fens. Take the A142 to the south-east to Ely (L), a town that stood on an island before the land was drained during the seventeenth and eighteenth centuries: there were marshlands all round Ely before the Fens were drained and the town could only be reached by boat or causeway. Many of the engineers brought in to build the dykes (an integral part of the drainage system) were Dutch craftsmen, already skilled at dyking the land. The Cathedral at Ely dominates the little town, and stands out for miles around in glorious silhouette on the flat fen landscape; the building was begun in 1080 and there is some fine carving to be seen in the choir. Try the White Hart Hotel on Market Street, an original building from the fifteenth century but with later additions; also the Lamb Hotel on Lynn Road, and the Club Hotel on Market Place which used to be a sporting club with a gym where boxers worked out.

From Ely take the A10 to the south and then turn right on to the A1123 to Houghton (H) a little village on the River Ouse where there are some lovely little cottages and a village green, and an old timber watermill which has been turned into a hostel. Visit the Three Jolly Butchers' Inn which has wall paintings from the seventeenth century. Stay on the A1123 to Hartford, then bear left on to the A141 to Huntingdon, the town which boasts both Cromwell and the diarist Samuel Pepys as grammar school pupils. The school has now been turned into a museum with a good selection of Cromwelliana, including his death mask. The George and The Falcon are two good inns in Huntingdon, the latter is supposed to have been the headquarters of Cromwell during the Civil War.

From Huntingdon take the A604 south-east past the town of Godmanchester (L), Huntingdon's twin town. Bear left on a loop road some four miles from Huntingdon to go through the charming village of Hemingford Grey (CH at Houghton). Follow the loop road back on to the A604 and turn left, south-west into Cambridge (LCH). If you wonder why the road is so straight, it is because the modern road was built on the course of an old Roman road, the Via Devana.

The first colleges of the ancient and renowned University of Cambridge were established in 1284. Modern Cambridge has been described as "perhaps the only true university town in England" and certainly the university buildings are the outstanding architectual feature of the town, especially Trinity College, where the library is by Christopher Wren and there are carvings by Grinling Gibbons; also King's College Chapel. The "Backs" are the landscaped lawns and gardens, behind the line of colleges, through which winds the River Cam. Northampton Street and Magdalene Street contain the best medieval houses and cottages with projecting upper stories. The Fitzwilliam Museum is worth a visit, with its fine collection of Egyptian, Greek and Roman antiquities. Have a pint at the Pickerel Inn in Magdalene Street: it looks as if it is part of Magdalene College—built in 1540, it was originally part of the monks' quarters. Two miles to the south-west of Cambridge is the peaceful little village of Grantchester where the poet Rupert Brooke lived and wrote before the First World War.

There are two route choices from Cambridge.

Cambridge to Long Melford (35 miles)

Take the A604 south-east from Cambridge to Linton, where you can wet your whistle either at the three hundred year old Dog and Duck, which has good vintage cider and a nice garden at the back, or at the five hundred year old Bell Inn where there oak beams, an open fireplace and good food.

Stay on the A604 through Haverhill (L) and bear left, not long after Haverhill, on to the A1092 for Clare, a lovely village of half-timbered cottages. Try the Swann Inn, which has been an alehouse since 1471 and has an oak tavern sign thought to be the oldest in England. Continue on the A1092 east into Long Melford (L), one of the prettiest of all English villages; this is the part of Suffolk which was *the* centre of the weaving industry in medieval England. Try the Bull Inn at Long Melford.

Cambridge to Long Melford via Norwich (130 miles)

The alternate route from Cambridge takes you east on the A45 from Cambridge and then left on the A11 through Newmarket which, set in open heathland, is the centre of English horse racing and the home of numerous stud farms; the first race on record took place in 1619 on a racecourse outside the town. Have a pint at the Rutland Arms Hotel or at the Georgian Jockey Club.

Bear left again after Newmarket on the A1065 through Brandon, Mundford and Hillsborough into Swaffham, a lovely if somewhat hectic market town with some good Georgian architecture. From Swaffham (L) take the A47 to East Dereham, where George Borrow, the enigmatic nineteenth century romantic

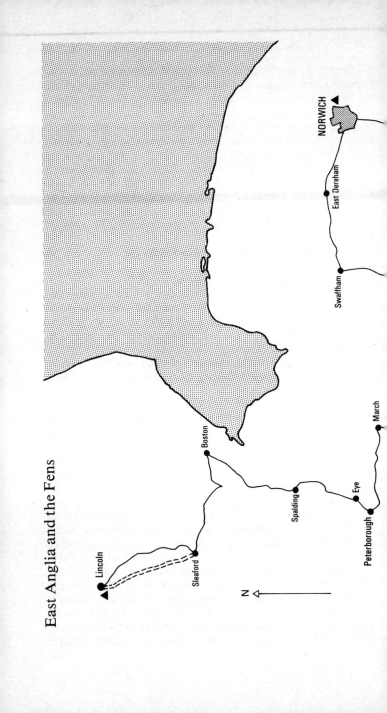

East Anglia and the Fens

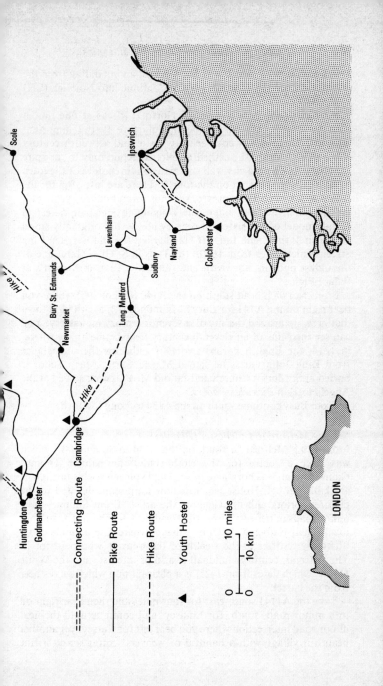

Scole

Ipswich

Hike

Bury St. Edmunds

Lavenham

Newmarket

Sudbury

Nayland

Long Melford

Colchester

Hike 1

Cambridge

Hike 1

Huntingdon

Godmanchester

===== Connecting Route

——— Bike Route

– – – Hike Route

▲ Youth Hostel

LONDON

10 miles

10 km

0

0

writer and linguist, was born; The George, an inn dating from the seventeenth century is worth a visit. Continue into Norwich (LH) on the A47.

Norwich is the county town of Norfolk; it was at one time a weaving centre, but now shoe manufacture is the important industry. There is a twelfth century castle and a twelfth century Norman cathedral. The cathedral spire is second only to the spire at Salisbury. The old city wall still exists on three sides of the town with the River Wensum on the fourth. There are lots of pubs: the Adam and Eve on Bishopsgate, which is seven hundred years old; the Blue Bell in Goat Lane; the Dolphin in Heigham Street (a rebuilt model of the sixteenth century house that originally stood on the site); the Lamb Inn, off Haymarket; the Old Barge in King Street (which dates from 1600); the Tuns in St Giles Gate (one of the oldest pubs in Norwich); and the White Lion in Martin's at Palace Plain.

From Norwich head south on the A140 to Scole (C) where you bear right on the A143 for Bury St Edmunds (L), a cathedral town that grew up around the site of a seventh century monastery. You can see the ruins of an eleventh century Benedictine abbey where, in 1214, the English barons swore to withdraw their allegiance from King John unless he signed Magna Carta. Mary Tudor is buried at St Mary's Church and fat old Mr Pickwick stayed at the Angel Hotel in *Pickwick Papers*.

From Bury continue south on the A134 to Long Melford.

Long Melford to Colchester (70 miles)

From Long Melford go south on the A134 to Sudbury (L) which was once a centre for the cloth trade; the painter Thomas Gainsborough was born here in 1727 and you can see his birthplace at Gainsborough House which is now a museum devoted to the pictures, prints and drawings of the artist. From Sudbury take minor roads north-east across the Heath to Lavenham (L), another lovely half-timbered Suffolk village where the church magnificently testifies to the wealth of the weavers who paid for it. The fifteenth century Guildhall is also of interest, and the White Horse, which dates from 1425, is a pleasant pub which serves beer from the barrel.

Take the A1141 south-east for four miles and then bear right on to a minor road, south, for Lindsey, and continue until the next minor road intersection where you bear left for Kersey, yet another beautiful village with a handful of weavers' cottages and a fine fifteenth century church. Follow the same minor road east to the junction with the A1141 where you turn right for Hadleigh. From Hadleigh travel east on the A1071 to Ipswich (L), an ancient market town and port at the head of the Orwell estuary, a hale and hearty town which still retains some medieval charm. Go to Tavern Street to see the Great White Horse Hotel where Charles Dickens stayed and which figures prominently in *Pickwick Papers*; try the fifteenth century Golden Lion Hotel in Cornhill; Manning's, a Victorian inn in Lion Street, dating from 1737; and the Margaret Catchpole Hotel, on Cliff Lane, which is named after a folk heroine of Suffolk.

From Ipswich take the A137 south towards Manningtree, but a mile or so north of Manningtree bear right for Flatford Mill on the River Stour, near East Bergholt. This is the countryside which has been immortalized in the paintings of John Constable. Constable (1776-1837) was born at the little village of East Bergholt. His father owned Flatford Mill where Constable worked for a year when he was eighteen. Follow the same minor road north-west to East Bergholt (L), where Constable was born, a village of half-timbered houses on the River Stour: try the Red Lion Inn on Gaston Street where draught cider is a speciality; this inn dates from 1700 and was surely visited by Constable.

Go north-west out of East Bergholt to the A12 and turn left for Stratford St Mary. From the north end of the village a minor road leads north-west along the River Stour and after two miles intersects with another minor road where you bear left for Stoke by Nayland, a quiet village. Continue by minor road south-west to Nayland (L) on the River Stour, a peaceful village with good fifteenth and sixteenth century houses. The fourteenth century Hart Hotel on the High Street, besides serving a good pint, is reputed to house the ghost of a woman who was murdered in Room Three; the footsteps of the soldier who murdered her are heard at night and a woman in black supposedly walks the halls.

From Nayland take the A134 south into the city of Colchester (LH), the oldest town in Britain. The first Roman city in Britain was founded here in 43 BC, parts of the old Roman wall still stand and the museum houses many Roman antiquities. Unfortunately the developers and town planners have been heavy-handed, destroying streets of lovely architecture but some historic buildings remain. Some of Constable's drawings are in the Minories Art Gallery, but more can be seen in the National Gallery in London.

There are rail connections from Colchester.

HIKING

East Anglia and the Fens bristle with good walking paths. This is a marvellous area just to buy an Ordnance Survey map in the 1:50,000 Series and explore on your own. To my mind the best areas where there are the most picturesque villages, such as Lavenham and Long Melford, are covered by maps 154 and 155 in the Ordnance Survey 1:50,000 Series. The paths described below are old Roman roads that have fallen into disuse in modern times, leaving fine, wide trackways which are easy for the walker to follow. There are no official long distance paths in this region.

TWO ROMAN ROADS

1. *The Via Devana: Cambridge to Haverhill (12 miles)*
This road was originally built by the Romans and stretches from Godmanchester through Cambridge to Haverhill. The section from Godmanchester to Cambridge is now a modern road on which you may have pedalled into Cambridge, but after Cambridge, the Via Devana is just a trackway leading south-east over the Gogmagog Hills and across Wandlebury Camp. The path does not pass through any villages, and it enters the county of Suffolk at Withersfield, just north of Haverhill where it disappears. You need Ordnance Survey map number 154 in the 1:50,000 Series for this hike.

2. *The Icknield Way*
This is a prehistoric trackway that goes much farther to the west and which you may have come across in other touring areas. Much of it today is paved road, but from Lackford on the River Lark, there is a four mile stretch of track that goes through King's Forest to Weatherhill Heath; here the Icknield Way forms the boundary of Elveden Park and two miles before Thetford all trace of it is lost. You need Ordnance Survey map number 144 in the 1:50,000 Series for this hike.

Further Information

In this book I have assumed that the traveller will want a mix of biking and hiking, and the book is organized as if one intended to do both. In some cases the bike and hike routes connect better than in others: sometimes a good hiking route begins at the terminus of a biking route, or even intersects that route, but not always. What about those people who are hiking and do not have a bike when they want to go biking; or, conversely, those who are biking and do not know where to leave their bike when hiking?

BIKE RENTAL and STORAGE

The Tourist Authorities (see page 221) publish up-to-date booklets listing all the places which rent out bikes, so, if you plan to rent a bike, contact in advance the Tourist Authorities which cover the areas you intend to tour. Alternatively, look under the Yellow Pages in the telephone directory: in tourist areas and near big cities, renting a bike should present no problem, but, obviously, the more remote the area the harder it will become to find a bike rental. However, be careful if you plan to rent a bike: some bike renters lend ten-speed bikes, others rent out only mini-bikes; also you take pot-luck with these bikes, so it is wise to look over the bike very thoroughly before renting it, checking the brakes and gears to see that they function properly.

Sometimes leaving your bike can be as big a problem as finding one. If you are staying at lodgings or in a hostel, it is best to leave it there, though of course this will depend on the co-operation of the person that runs the B and B or the warden of the hostel.

Always offer to pay: you will probably never have to, but it makes your request legitimate. The best place to leave your bike, however, is at a railway station in the Left Luggage. There is a standard charge for a bike which is left for up to two days, on the same conditions that apply to other large articles, and, in some cases, British Rail accepts liability; there are also weekly, monthly and quarterly rates, but bikes are left at the owner's risk. Garages, storage companies and car parks will sometimes store bikes; also places that follow no general rule; at Avebury, for example, not far from the Ridgeway Path, a lady at the car park just across the road from the entrance to the stone circles said that she would let anyone leave their bike in her back yard while they hiked the Ridgeway. I then told her that I was writing a guide book, she still graciously upheld her offer, but she looked rather worried and asked, "You don't think they'll come in the hundreds though, do you?"

SOME INFORMATION FOR BIKERS
FROM OTHER COUNTRIES

Rent or Buy

I would not necessarily advise visitors to Britain to bring their own bikes. Although bikes are considered part of the forty-two pounds baggage allowance on flights, you will have a few pounds of clothing and anything over the baggage allowance is payable depending upon the flight distance. But if you travel light and are only planning on biking (so that you will not have to pay for storage for a long time when not biking), it *might* be wise to bring your bike. If you do not bring a bike with you, you will have either to buy or rent one in Britain. Second-hand bikes are almost impossible to find. You will not get as good a bike when renting as when buying, so I recommend that anyone planning to bike for more than a month should buy a moderately priced bike in Britain. For the casual biker, someone wanting to bike for only one or two weeks here and there, the best thing would be to rent.

If you buy a new bike, you can be sure of selling it back to a dealer after you finish your touring for at least half-price. If you sell it to a private party, which involves a little more hassle, you could get much more on a resale. Advertise in a local paper or put a *For Sale* sign on the bike towards the end of your journey. You should have no trouble selling in a few days as good touring model bikes are a very popular second-hand purchase and usually hard to find. You may have more difficulty with odd bikes, for example, super tall bikes or heavy, old uprights; easiest to resell is the lightweight ten-speed.

A word of caution to those planning to begin their biking in Southern Ireland: Southern Ireland has a value-added tax on everything imported, and as there are no bicycle manufacturers in Southern Ireland, you can expect to pay from five to thirty percent more on a bike in Ireland than you would in Britain. Also, bikes exported to Ireland are not always the most modern. It is also almost impossible to find second-hand bikes in Southern Ireland; so, if you do not take a bike with you, it is better either to rent, or to buy a bike with the intention of reselling it before you leave.

Traffic Laws

Bicycles are subject to general vehicular laws. The most important of these is that you ride on the left in the British Isles. It is said that this curious custom began in the day when the highwaymen made the roads unsafe: most people, being right-handed, wished to ride on the left so as to meet any oncoming villain with their sword or pistol arm at the ready on the inside of the road. Others say that left-hand driving is just another example of British eccentricity; but, whatever the reason it can be hard for foreign visitors to get used to, especially when turning a corner at a junction.

Bikes must be equipped with two independent brakes: at front and back. At night—i.e. a half hour after sunset and half hour before sunrise—a bike must carry a front white light, a back red light, and a back red reflector. There are other minutiae regulating the diameter size of lights and their distance from the ground, but most bikes comply with these regulations as a matter of course.

There are two traffic signs that pertain only to bikes: a square blue sign with a white bike in the centre designates a bike path; a black bike on a white background, sometimes with a red slash through the bike, means that no bikes are allowed.

When you bike in the cities, be sure to obey the one-way signs, though it is always a temptation to take the quickest way. The Irish police especially can be tough with tourist bikers in their cities. Each policeman has a different signal for stop and go at city junctions and you must watch them fairly carefully.

Road Classification

The roads in Britain are classified thus: "M" is a motorway, marked blue on maps, and is the only road from which cyclists are forbidden; "A" roads are main roads, marked red on maps, and best avoided as much as possible by cyclists for they are usually quite busy. "B" roads are main local routes, some are busy, some are not; and then there are the minor or unclassified routes which are the best for biking—the quiet and pastoral back lanes you will love. These are usually marked yellow on maps.

Irish roads are similarly classified, though different letters are used: "T" and "N" roads are main roads; "L" roads are secondary routes like "B" roads in Britain.

Bikes may not be used on footpaths, but they may be used on paths broad enough to be designated as bridleways, where horse riding is also allowed, though these bridleways may prove rough going in places.

ACCOMMODATION

Whether biking or hiking, you are going to have to stay somewhere at night, and there are several lodging possibilities. The most typical are the Bed and Breakfasts: B and B. These are small, family-run houses providing a good inexpensive night's lodging and a hearty egg and bacon breakfast. In the English and Irish countryside there is another particularly pleasant type of accommodation: farmhouses. These farmhouses are often located in out of the way places, and are functioning farms which rent out a couple of rooms like a B and B. They are quiet, homely and comfortable, and you will eat some very good food for there will be fresh eggs and home-churned butter. It is usually possible to have an evening meal at a farmhouse, depending on how far removed it is from civilization. It will cost about the same as a B and B. There are also inns, which are often old buildings with real charm: they will cost you more than a B and B, but are worth the expense once in a while. You will find one or other of these forms of accommodation in most places, or at least a higher-priced hotel. It is only in the busy months of July and August that you need really worry about getting a night's lodgings or whether you need reservations.

Another inexpensive and omnipresent form of accommodation is the youth hostel. There are four hundred hostels in the British Isles, and they can be a life-saver: look for the sign with a tree and a little hut stencilled on. You can get a dormitory-style night's lodging at a hostel and, depending on the grade of the hostel and the age of the hosteller, it will be very cheap. Anyone from five years old to ninety-five can stay at a hostel: I have met a retired couple in their seventies from Melbourne, and ten-year-old students from Tokyo. Most hostels provide meals: breakfast, dinner and a lunch packet. They also have kitchens for members' use, free of charge, and also a small shop (except in the Republic of Ireland) for the purchase of staples. As many of the hostels are away from towns, be sure you can buy food at the hostel before leaving any villages with shops. When you stay at a hostel you must have what is called a sheet sleeping bag; these can be purchased at most hostels or, alternatively, you can rent one at each hostel. The bags protect the hostel blankets and pillows. Ordinary sleeping bags cannot be used. Hostels usually close early at night—ten-thirty to eleven p.m.—and are closed during the day from about ten a.m. till five p.m. Everyone has a "duty" to do in the morning: sweeping up, cleaning the wash basins, etc, and this is OK because everyone is doing it.

A room at a B and B or a bed at a hostel is not difficult to find in May or June and September or October; but during July and August, if you do not have reservations, and if there is more than one of you, then you can be sure that you will spend half the day worrying about where you are going to sleep that night, and the other half hunting for a place. Competition is worst at the hostels where people start queuing two or three hours before opening time: for an organization developed to promote goodwill between people, this is a situation ripe for international incidents; but worst of all, you have got to waste a couple of hours waiting (maybe in the rain) and often not even knowing if you will get a bed or not. B and Bs can be almost as bad, especially in such tourist favourites as the Lake District and Cornwall; and especially if you arrive at your destination after five p.m.

You *can* reserve accommodation ahead of time: there are accommodation books published by the Tourist Authorities (see page 221); the Cyclists' Touring Club and the Ramblers' Association also both publish, for their members, books listing thousands of B and Bs all over the British Isles. There are also Tourist Boards all over the British Isles, which for a small fee will find you lodgings for the night and will also help you to book ahead. Look for the green-trimmed signs with an "I" in the middle which will direct you to the local Tourist Information Office. Ireland's Bord Failte is much the best of any of the Tourist

Boards, being connected with all other Boards in the country and able to tell you exactly what is available where. You can book ahead at hostels for the holiday months. When joining the Y.H.A. (Youth Hostels Association, see page 220), ask for booking coupons, and when you have planned your tour well enough to know where you will be when, write to each hostel early enough to get a response and a receipt. You can also order a sheet sleeping bag from the YHA, and a handbook of all the hostels in various parts of the world, plus maps showing their location.

Camping

B and Bs and youth hostels are two forms of fairly civilized accommodation; but really the best alternative for the biker, and almost a necessity for the hiker, is camping. The biker or hiker who carries camping equipment is independent—he has a choice, there is all the outdoors in which to sleep, or there is the comfort of a bed under a roof. By carrying camping equipment you can avoid having to become just one of the crowd of tired and hungry bodies who besiege hotel people during the high season. For the hiker there is often no choice but to camp: there will be some nights on the long-distance routes when the nearest roof will be several miles from the path. Camping equipment will take up half your pack, but it will be the most valuable half. Throughout the tours I have indicated where there are public camp-sites: these are very handy for the camper because they have toilet and bathing facilities; but I would not advise their use solely, for these campsites also cater for caravans and they can be very crowded and noisy. Several guides are published each year (for example by the British Tourist Authority, see page 221) which list camping facilities with maps of their locations.

There are many places in the British Isles where you can camp without difficulty and avoid the official camping sites (which are not always cheap). There are areas of open country, such as moorland, where you can pitch a tent; but if there is only private farmland available, ask the farmer if you can camp on his land for the night; assure him that you will leave the campsite clean and offer to pay. The payment will rarely be accepted. Always leave a site clean and burn or pick up litter especially if you are on private land.

You might want to buy an "International Camping Carnet" which allows the holder to camp at the official sites of various touring clubs around the world. The card also provides a limited insurance of your camping equipment and can act as a good form of identification, especially for farmers whom you would like to impress favourably so as to camp in their field for the night. You can purchase this card through the Cyclists' Touring Club (see page 220).

Two other organizations may prove helpful: the Association of Cycle and Lightweight Campers, and the Camping Club of Great Britain and Ireland. Both organizations have camping site lists for sale and may be able to advise you further on aspects of camping in the British Isles (see page 220).

PUBLIC TRANSPORT

The tours given in this book may be taken together to make a grand tour of the whole of the British Isles; but it is very seldom that the biker and the hiker will never be able to cover the distances between touring areas by self-propulsion. Public transport will have to be used at some time or other.

Public transport is not cheap, though buses are always less expensive than trains; however, bicycles cannot be carried on buses except in Ireland (on buses that have room). In Ireland bikes cost a quarter of the second class train fare; by bus, and whether bikes are taken on the bus or not depends on the mood of the driver and the amount of baggage already being carried, a bike costs the same regardless of the passenger fare. It is usually better to go by train if you are transporting a bike. On British rail and ferry services, bikes cost half of the second class fare.

There are many fare reductions on public transport in the British Isles. Some fare reductions are only available to visitors from other countries who should write for up-to-date information to the British Railways Board (see page 221), or check with their travel agent. There are other reductions on train fares in Britain which apply to everyone: you can buy the Rover Season Ticket for one week's unlimited travel and day-return tickets can also be purchased very cheaply—sometimes they are cheaper than a normal one-way ticket, so check on this reduction even if you are only going one way.

The Coachmaster Bus Pass allows you unlimited distance at a much cheaper rate than trains (but no bikes carried): tickets can be purchased from National Travel Limited at Victoria Coach Station.

Bus tours can be very cheap, especially in Scotland, but they are designed for tourists wanting an organized tour. The cost of the outward journey on one of these round trips is often less than the cost of using public transport, but if you join a tour with your pack you will probably not be popular and you may not even be allowed on the coach, so this is only a last resort suggestion for when you have really run out of time and money.

In Ireland you can buy the Rambler Ticket, which gives you fifteen days of unlimited travel; and for about twenty-five per cent more you can also use the national CIE bus service with the same stipulations. The Irish also have eight-day tickets for rail alone, and for combined rail and bus travel. These tickets may be purchased in Ireland at the CIE train and bus stations.

Storage

There are places in most large cities where you can leave your excess baggage for a moderate rate. Most British railway stations no longer accept baggage on a long-term basis, so it is better to find a removal and storage company for long-term deposits; Bishop and Sons' Depositories Limited (see page 221) in London is near Victoria Station, which is the most convenient railway station in London for leaving baggage, as it is the terminus for trains from Gatwick Airport and from the Continent, via Dover or Folkestone, and also only a short ride on the Underground from anywhere in the city.

PASSES

If you fulfill the requirements, an International Student Identity Card is worth having. You must be a full-time student and under thirty years of age when you apply. If you have one of these cards you can get reduced fares on planes and trains all over the world; you also get free admission to most museums.

There are also season tickets to museums, public gardens and country houses which, depending on your likes and dislikes and whether or not you already have a student card, it may be worth your while to have. Ask at museums or at National Trust Properties.

CLUBS

There are two clubs well worth joining in England that will give the real afficionado much in-depth information. One club is for bikers, the other for hikers.

The Cyclists' Touring Club

The Cyclists' Touring Club is almost one hundred years old. Its avowed aim is "to promote, assist and protect the use of bicycles, tricycles, and other similar vehicles on the public roads and rights of way"; but it does much more. Among its services to members is an extensive library of bike routes and touring areas, copies of which are sold at minimal prices. Some of these tour maps have information sheets accompanying them, describing interesting sites along the route. The CTC also maintains an extensive selection of road maps in the Ordnance Survey and Bartholomew series (see page 218). The maps are sold to members at a very fair price. The CTC handbook, which is available to members, has a list of three thousand B and Bs, plus the addresses of bike repairers in all regions. The handbook is also chock full of other valuable information regarding biking, as well as transport timetables: all invaluable information for cycle tourists. The CTC also publishes an illustrated magazine on biking every two months; and offers the services of a legal aid to members and also various insurance policies, both in the case of road accident. The CTC is affiliated with other clubs and offers members such purchases as the International Camping Carnet.

I would advise you to join the CTC sometime before you plan to start touring, so that you can really make use of the tour-planning services of the club. The people at CTC are a friendly lot and anxious to help with any question about biking in Britain and on the Continent (they have a full range of maps and routes for the Continent).

The Ramblers' Association

The emphasis of the Ramblers' Association is mainly on political action to protect the environment; but by protecting the environment, it thereby directly aids its members who walk in the said environment. The club states that public access to the land should be a legal right, and in the 1930s and 40s it fought to persuade Parliament that ordinary folk should have the right to roam mountain and moorland country. The National Parks and

Access to the Countryside Act of 1949 conceded this principle and empowered county councils to make agreements, or failing agreements, orders, giving the public freedom to roam on uncultivated land. The Ramblers' Association also protects existing public rights of way, in the form of access paths across a farmer's land, by regularly walking many miles of such path to see if any obstructions to the path have been made. It is interesting to know this history, for once you are hiking and using these access paths, you will appreciate the tight situations that sometimes develop between the farmers and groups such as The Ramblers' who want to provide a public right of way across private land; so take care when using these rights of way, stick to the paths and close gates after you, for it is all a delicate balance of compromise.

The Ramblers' Association has a huge bibliography of literature in the field of walking and hiking. There are numerous works available describing walks in various parts of Britain, and they are detailed almost to foot-by-foot descriptions. The Ramblers' has lists of these publications together with prices, and where they may be purchased. In addition to this excellent bibliography, The Ramblers' also has a large collection of Ordnance Survey maps in the 1:50,000 series (see page 218). What is unique about this collection is that The Ramblers' lends these maps out to their members; and since each map is very detailed and covers only a small area this library can be a good source and worth the membership money paid. The Ramblers' also publishes a quarterly magazine containing good articles on hiking skills and on the environment. The club also has a helpful handbook which lists B and Bs around Britain and bus schedules. Unlike the CTC, The Ramblers' does not have a library of proposed hiking routes. They will direct you to the right agency or publication if asked about specific hiking areas, but the preparation of these routes is not part of their service. There are three organizations that do arrange hikes, walking holidays and long distance walks, which include lodging, and are led by a competent outdoors person; they are: The Countrywide Holidays Association; Holiday Fellowship; and The Youth Hostels Association; (see page 220).

THE COUNTRYSIDE AND MOUNTAIN CODE

1. Respect private property and keep to the paths when going through estates and farmland. Avoid where possible climbing over

walls and fences and close gates that you open. Do not leave litter.

2. Be careful not to disturb sheep in the lambing season (April to May), and avoid deer-stalking and grouse-shooting country during these seasons (usually August to October). If in doubt, enquire from local farmers or keepers before going on the hills. Keep dogs under control on the hills.

3. In forests, keep to paths, avoid smoking and do not light fires. Avoid damaging young trees in newly planted areas.

4. Plan your climb carefully, taking account of the experience and fitness of the party, the prevailing weather and the weather forecast. Watch out for the weather in the mountains, especially in Snowdonia and in the Scottish Highlands—weather here changes exceedingly fast and you can easily become lost if wandering off the main path when the mists come rolling in. Allow plenty of time for the climb in daylight hours and plan the route beforehand on a map.

5. Be properly equipped for your climb, and carry adequate food.

6. Leave a note in the hotel where you are staying, or with the police or other responsible person, or, failing that, in your car or tent, of the names of the party, the objective, the route up and down, and the expected time of return.

7. Be prepared to turn back if the weather turns bad, or if any member of the party is going very slowly or is exhausted. The party should keep together, especially in misty weather.

8. Be particularly careful in the descent, especially if the route is unknown to you. If in doubt, go down by your uphill route. Do not run downhill; a sprained ankle might mean a rescue team call-out.

9. In the event of an accident requiring a rescue team, at least one person should stay with the injured climber while one or two go down for help. If there are only two in the party, the injured climber should be left with all the spare clothing, food, whistle and torch while his companion goes for help. The person descending to the valley should inform the police as quickly as possible.

Warning

Exposure is a common danger to the hill walker and lowlands hiker alike. It can happen even in midsummer and is usually caused by getting wet in windy weather. The body becomes severely chilled—blow on your wet hand and you will get an idea of what happens. This can happen at any time in the mountains if you are ill-prepared, and also in the lowlands, particularly on the moors where there are few wind breaks.

One of the best ways to prevent exposure is to have adequate clothing, especially a good, really waterproof rain jacket or a cape with a hood. An exhausted person is more prone to exposure than someone who is still fit and in good shape. Wearing too much clothing unnecessarily, especially waterproofs, can speed exhaustion. Take food on your walk and keep your energy up while out of doors. Watch for weather changes and avoid hiking in bad weather if it is at all possible. Do not go hiking if you are unwell.

The early warning signs of exposure are: unexpected or unreasonable behaviour; stumbling and mental deterioration; complaints of cold and tiredness; pallor, and shivering which stops as the person becomes colder.

The best thing you can do if you notice these signs, is to get to cover. Immediate rest and shelter is needed. Keep the person warm to stop further heat loss; give hot drinks and sugar or glucose in some form. Do *not* give alcohol or rub the limbs in an attempt to improve circulation. Do *not* provide localized heat, such as a hot water bottle, and do not let the patient walk even if he or she says they are feeling better. Go for help, and if you must leave the person, be sure they are well covered and write down your map reference point.

Heat exhaustion and sunstroke are also a danger so wear a hat, drink salted drinks and stay out of the sun in the hottest times of the day. Some of the first signs of heat exhaustion are headache and nausea, a florid complexion and cramps; eventually perspiration will cease and the person will collapse. This can be treated by getting the person out of the sun and removing the outer clothing to help cooling. Put wet towels on to limbs and head and give water that has a half teaspoon of salt to every pint. If the person becomes unconscious, get help.

MAPS

Whether you are biking or hiking you will need maps. The Ordnance Survey in Great Britain publishes excellent maps of England, Wales and Scotland to many different scales. Their *Route Planning Map* at a scale of about one inch to ten miles covers the whole of Great Britain, showing the South on one side of the sheet and the North on the other. It is specially designed for planning routes in advance and is a good reference map for travellers and particularly for bikers. The Ordnance Survey also publish a series of fifteen maps of Great Britain at a scale of four miles to the inch called *Quarter-Inch Maps*.

Bartholomew, the Scottish firm of map-makers publish a series of three route planning maps called *Tourist Route Maps* at a scale of nine miles to one inch; they are of *Southern England* (including Wales), *Northern England* and *Scotland*. They also publish a series of *Touring Maps* at a scale of twelve miles to the inch. These have the advantage to the biker of using contour colouring to indicate gradient. Bartholomew also publish a series at a scale of half an inch to one mile. These are called the "biker's friend" because of the detailed contour gradients that they show as well as all the unclassified backroads—those country lanes away from all the traffic which are such a joy to pedal on. However this series will be gradually phased out to be replaced by the new *1:100,000 Series* of maps at a scale of 1.6 miles to the inch. The main drawback of these maps, for the biker who plans on long distance touring, is that each map covers such a small area. There are sixty-two sheets in the series and the long distance biker would have to use a different map every day. The time to use these maps is when you discover a particular area which you want to explore thoroughly.

The Ordnance Survey publish many maps for the hiker. The *1:50,000 Series,* at a scale of about one and a quarter inches to one mile, is probably the most useful. These maps have a grid reference system which makes the finding of locations easier, and which the hiker must use on some of the cross country walks in this book. There are 204 sheets in the series and each map covers an area of about 620 square miles. The Ordnance Survey also publish the *1:25,000 Series,* at a scale of two and a half inches to the mile, and these are very useful for areas that you wish to explore in depth or for routes that are difficult to follow. Both the 1:50,000 Series and the 1:25,000 Series mark public footpaths with broken or dotted lines. In England and Wales public paths are marked in red, and paths the status of which is private or unknown are marked in black—on these there is no guaranteed right of way. This information is not given on maps of Scotland as Scottish county councils are not required to record public rights of way; however Scotland has no operative law of trespass—broken lines on Scottish maps denote footpaths, but not whether or not they are public. These maps show contours and gradient and there are many symbols on them, so be sure to read the legend thoroughly in order to get full use of them. In addition to the 1:50,000 and 1:25,000 Series, the Ordnance Survey publish a series of one-inch to the mile *Tourist Maps* which cover very popular tourist areas. These give extra information, useful to tourists—for example: the location of view points and National Park Information Centres—and, in addition to the usual contour lines, these maps show relief by shading.

Southern Ireland

The Ordnance Survey in Ireland publish a *General Map of Ireland* at a scale of nine miles to the inch which shows "T", "L" and other roads as well as the distance in miles between towns, scenic roads and views, youth hostels, airports, etc. There is also a series of five maps at a scale of a quarter of an inch to one mile; these show gradient and topography. There is a half-inch to the mile series and a one inch to the mile series for the hiker.

Bartholomew publish a quarter-inch series of five maps called *Travel Maps* which have a contour colouring to show gradient. Bartholomew also publish a touring map at a scale of twelve miles to one inch.

USEFUL ADDRESSES

Clubs and Organizations

The Cyclists' Touring Club (CTC), 69 Meadrow, Godalming, Surrey GU7 3HS

The Ramblers' Association, 1/4 Crawford Mews, York Street, London W1H 1PT

The Camping Club of Great Britain and Ireland Limited, 11 Grosvenor Place, London SW1W 0EY

The Association of Cycle and Lightweight Campers, Secretary's address: 30 Napier Way, Wembley, Middlesex HA0 4UA; *or:* Sinnott House, Birch Street, Southport, Merseyside PR8 5EP.

Youth Hostels Association (YHA)

England and Wales: Trevelyan House, 8 St Stephens Hill, St Albans, Hertfordshire AL1 2DY; *or:* 29 John Adam Street, London WC2N 6JE

Scotland: 7 Glebe Crescent, Stirling

Eire: 39 Mountjoy Square, Dublin

The Countrywide Holidays Association, Birch Heys, Cromwell Range, Manchester M14 6HW

Holiday Fellowship, 142 Great North Way, Hendon, London NW4 1EG

National Parks

National Parks' Headquarters, Bank House, High Street, Windermere, Cumbria LA23 1AF

Exmoor National Park, Exmoor House, Delverton, Somerset TA22 9LH

Dartmoor National Park, Devon County Council, County Hall, Exeter, Devon EX2 4QA

Brecon Beacons National Park, Glamorgan Street, Brecon, Powys LD3 7DW

Pembrokeshire Coast National Park, Dyfed County Council, County Offices, Haverfordwest, Dyfed SA61 1QR

Snowdonia National Park, The Old School House, Maentwrog, Blaenau Ffestiniog, Gwynedd LL41 4HW

Lake District National Park, Brockhole, Near Windermere, Cumbria LA23 1W

Yorkshire Dales National Park, Colvend, Hebden Road, Grassington, Skipton, North Yorkshire BD23 5LB

Northumberland National Park, Bede House, All Saints Office Centre, Newcastle-upon-Tyne NE1 2DH

Peak District National Park, Peak Park Planning Board, Aldern House, Baslow Road, Bakewell, Derbyshire DE4 1AE

Tourist Boards (for correspondence only)

English Tourist Board and London Tourist Board, 4 Grosvenor Gardens, London SW1W 0DU

Scottish Tourist Board, 23 Ravelston Terrace, Edinburgh EH4 3EU

Welsh Tourist Board, Welcome House, Llandaff, Cardiff CF5 2YZ

Bord Failte Eireann (Republic of Ireland), Baggot Street Bridge, Dublin 2

Tourist Information Offices (for help with lodging etc.)

London Tourist Centre, Platform 15, Victoria Station, London

British Tourist Authority, 64 St James Street, London SW1 1NF

Irish Tourist Office, 14 Upper O'Connel Street, Dublin 1; *or:* 51 Dawson Street, Dublin 2

Edinburgh Tourist Office, 5 Waverley Bridge, Edinburgh EH4 3EU

Miscellaneous

The Countryside Commission, John Dower House, Crescent Place, Cheltenham, Gloucestershire GL50 3RA

British Railways Board, 222 Marylebone Road, London NW1 6JJ

Ordnance Survey, Romsey Road, Maybush, Southampton SO9 4DH

Ordnance Survey, Phoenix Park, Dublin

John Bartholomew and Sons Limited, Duncan Street, Edinburgh EH9 1TA

Bishop and Sons' Depositories Limited, 10-12 Belgrave Road, London SW1 1QE

The Irish Traditional Music Society, 6 Harcourt Street, Dublin 2

BOOKS AND PAMPHLETS

Biking

England by Bicycle by Frederick Anderson, David and Charles

Cycle Touring in Europe by Peter Knottley, Constable

Explore the Cotswolds by Bicycle, British Cycling Bureau

Cycle Touring by Robin Adshead, Oxford Illustrated Press

Hiking

The Oldest Road—An Exploration of the Ridgeway by J. R. L. Anderson and Fay Godwin, Wildwood House

Hill Walking in Snowdonia by E. G. Rowland, Welsh Tourist Board

Walking in Wales, Welsh Tourist Board

Scotland for Hill Walking, Scottish Tourist Board

Scottish Hill Tracks—Old Highways and Drove Roads by D. G. Moir, Bartholomew

Walks in the Cotswolds by Ronald Kershaw and Brian Robson, Shire Publications Limited·

Walking the Pennine Way by Alan P. Binns, Gerrard Publications

The Cleveland Way and *The Pennine Way,* HMSO Publications

Coastal Paths of the Southwest by Edward C. Pyatt, David and Charles

Cornwall Coast Path, Cornwall Tourist Board

The Shell Book of Offa's Dyke Path by Frank Noble, Queen Anne Press
The Offa's Dyke Path by Arthur Roberts, Ramblers Association
The Pembrokeshire Coast Path, Countryside Commission
Isle of Skye Handbook, Scottish Mountaineering Club
No Through Road—The AA Book of Country Walks, Drive Publications

The Ramblers' Association has a large bibliography in the field of walking and hiking.

Camping
The Backpackers' Handbook by Derrick Booth, Hale
Backpacking by Peter Lumley, Teach Yourself Books
Backpacking in Britain by Robin Adshead and Derrick Booth, Oxford Illustrated Press
Britain: Caravan and Camping Sites, British Tourist Authority

General Books and Pamphlets
Inns of Britain, British Tourist Authority
Hotels and Restaurants in Britain, British Tourist Authority
Egon Ronay's Pubs and Tourist Sights in Britain, British Tourist Authority
Snowdonia National Park by William Condry, Collins
Geology and Scenery in England and Wales by A. E. Trueman, Penguin
Collins Pocket Guide to British Birds by Fitter and Richardson, Collins
A Field Guide to the Birds of Britain and Europe by Peterson, Mountfort and Hollom, Collins
The Hamlyn Guide to Birds of Britain and Europe by Bertel Bruun, Hamlyn
British Wild Flowers by I. Hutchinson, David and Charles
Camelot and the Vision of Albion by Geoffrey Ashe, Panther
The Quest for Arthur's Britain by Geoffrey Ashe, Paladin
View Over Atlantis by John Michell, Sphere
Official Guide to Farmhouses, Hotels and Guesthouses, Irish Tourist Board
Antiquities of the Irish Countryside by Sean O'Riordain, University Paperbacks, Methuen
Brendan Behan's Ireland by Brendan Behan, Hutchinson
A Book of Ireland by Frank O'Connor, Fontana
The Great Hunger by Cecil Woodham Smith, New English Library